How to *Actually* Live Longer Vol.1

CHRISTIAN YORDANOV

The information in this book is intended for educational purposes only. It is based on the research and professional experience of the author and should not be taken as professional medical advice, nor is it to be used as a substitute for medical care. For medical advice, always consult your physician and get their approval before implementing dietary changes or beginning any nutritional supplements. All efforts have been made to assure the accuracy of the information contained in this book as of the date of publication. The author and publisher specifically disclaim all responsibility for any liability, loss or risk, personal or otherwise, that is incurred as a consequence, directly or indirectly, of the use and application of the contents of this book. The publisher is not responsible for websites (or their content) that are not owned by the publisher.

ISBN: 978-1-9163930-2-8

First Edition

To Ingrida, with all my love.

Contents

Introduction

My oldest grandparent lived until the age of eighty-four with barely any knowledge of what even vitamins or minerals were. That is nine whole years longer than the current life expectancy in my home country of Bulgaria, and decades longer than what it was when she was born. I could not find data from the 1930s, but in 1950, the life expectancy for a Bulgarian was only 59 years.

Grandma did incredibly well in terms of lifespan, but by other metrics, the last years of her life were torture. She had several strokes and was on multiple drugs for three decades. Like most of her generation, she was hardy, having been raised on home-grown organic food in a world devoid of plastics and industrial pollution. I remember her working multiple jobs even after retiring. She was ever cheery, never complained, and always ready to help you out.

But taking care of my granddad during his health deterioration destroyed her health. Having worked as a carpenter, he was active throughout his younger years. However, after moving to an apartment in the city, poring over books and watching television replaced tending a garden and doing endless jobs around the house. He became increasingly sedentary in his last years; eventually, he found it hard to get out of his armchair. Grandma would bring him food, help him to the bathroom, and look after him in every way. When he fell to the floor, she somehow mustered up the strength to help him up. After granddad's passing, her health started deteriorating precipitously; the heartache of losing her mate pushed her over the edge.

Though she will never know it, grandma played a major role in my life's trajectory. Witnessing her slow and painful degeneration was the final wake-up call I needed to get my act together. Having recently met the woman I knew was to become my wife, my priorities were suddenly changing—but the gravity of my situation was setting in. The damage I had inflicted on myself during my twenties was unrivalled, except perhaps by the most misguided and irresponsible amongst us, and fear and regret were tormenting me.

We all do dumb things when we're young, but I would have made the Olympic team. When others mentioned my self-destructive lifestyle, I'd sometimes quip, "Don't worry, my body is a temple—a Temple of Doom!" with an arrogant air of indestructibility that is all too common in the youth. From dropping out of college to work as a bartender, drinking, smoking, partying, not sleeping, eating horrendous food (if we can even call much of what I ate food), breaking a leg, two years of working night shift, the list of poor choices is longer than my arm.

My complete disregard for the future impact of my actions was now starting to catch up with me. Though I had no apparent health problems yet (other than aches from the injuries and ample grey hair), my most pressing worry was my fertility and whether I could have healthy children. And if I did, whether I would live long enough to see them grow up; much less to see my grandkids.

But even if I was fortunate enough to survive to old age, I did not want to end up a burden on my loved ones, like my grandad was on my grandma, and like she later became on my mom and aunt. Nor did I want to see my future wife degenerate into her old age. Her professional ballet career had taken a serious toll on her health, and the medical system was now only making her worse. To put it in perspective, her doctors put her on antibiotics *four* times during our first year together. Because this often inappropriately used intervention frequently leads to fungal overgrowth, she was back at the doctor's office. How did they decide to "treat" the problem this time? By putting her on birth control, of course! As you do...

I can't tell you how appalled and frustrated I was. Everywhere I turned, people were unwell, but the system was, at best, useless in helping them. As a quick example, my mother suffered from irritable bowel system (IBS) for thirteen years and her doctor did *nothing* to help her during that time. It was time to take responsibility and find the solutions that had to be outside of the obviously broken conventional medical paradigm.

I knew plenty of people lived disease-free lives well into their nineties—I just had to figure out whether it came down to their superior genetics or if we could exert a significant influence on the ageing process. Since you're holding this book, it's clear that genetics are not the dominant factor. In fact, it's mostly our daily habits that play the biggest role in how quickly we degenerate. And while today I have more grey hair and metal bolts and plates in my body than I'd like, I believe the dysfunction that could be reversed, has been, and my metabolic health now rivals that of many people 20 years younger. However, this does not bring me joy, but consternation. I could not keep the information I learned to myself; not with the rampaging chronic disease crisis ruining our loved ones' and neighbours' lives. I was glad I could help my mother resolve her IBS fully in several months and that my wife enjoyed a two-year stretch where she didn't fall sick even once, but it was evident there was more work to be done.

The intense desire to undo the damage I inflicted on myself turned into a passion that is now my job. My specialties are in helping clients navigate chronic and complex conditions, and assisting those who are proactively seeking to invest in their long-term health. With my first book, *Autism Wellbeing Plan: How to Get Your Child Healthy*, I sought to teach parents of autistic children about the hidden metabolic challenges their kids face and how to identify and address them. After a young member of my family was suspected to be on the spectrum and witnessing the woefully inadequate support parents of autistic children receive, I felt the need for this detour.

Of course, my quest to uncover the keys of health optimisation and longevity continued in parallel; it is now time to share with you the most impactful nuggets of wisdom I've gleaned through the thousands of hours of research and experimentation, and my clinical experience. I take solace that while I cannot help my family members who have passed or do not care to listen to my message, I can pay it forward and play my role in repairing the damage the modern world and its associated systems have caused to our collective health. The task is gargantuan, but like eating an elephant, we eat it one bite at a time. Or in this case, one person at a time (no biting or eating will be involved, I promise). That person is you, and I am honoured you chose this book as your guide.

If you read and apply the information in this series, you will live longer *and* you will have more life in your years. You will age slower and stave off degeneration for longer than you would have otherwise. Unless a piano falls on your head, of course—nothing we can do about chance. Further, you can accomplish this increased life- and healthspan without fasting, restricting calories, avoiding meat, eating lots of vegetables, tons of exercise, or subjecting yourself to stressful activities like cold plunges or whatever other nonsense permeates the mainstream this week.

How can I state such bold claims? It will make sense when you **understand the mechanisms through which the body ages and becomes dysfunctional**. For now, let's see how the older you will differ from the younger you. When researchers compare blood markers and other anthropometric measures of people in their twenties to those in their seventies *without* diabetes, cancer, or untreated diseases of the heart, thyroid, liver, and kidneys, they find that the older adults usually have a combination of the following:

- More inflammation in their body
- Reduced antioxidant status
- More DNA damage
- Increased stress hormones
- Lower levels of the protective hormones
- Increased insulin resistance
- Poorer cognitive function
- Less muscle mass and strength
- Increased fat mass

For an example from the literature, here is what one study found:

> …compared to healthy young adults, older humans have severely elevated oxidative stress, glutathione [antioxidant] deficiency, impaired mitochondrial function, increased inflammation, insulin resistance and endothelial dysfunction, and lower muscle strength and mental cognition.[1]

Do you want to know the "secret"? Most of the above are easy to improve—even in old age—with a few supplements and dietary and lifestyle changes. But if you start early, you can avoid most of these "features" of ageing. Yes, growing old is inevitable, but growing sick and decrepit is entirely optional. The key is to have the right information and apply it consistently.

Here is the even better news: you are about to start learning how to mitigate the factors that age you prematurely and how to support your body's defence and repair systems. Now, imagine you started addressing these factors earlier in life, say, in your forties, fifties, or even sixties. If you started today—how much better off would you be in six months, or six years? How would it change the trajectory of your life and health? I'll tell you how: immensely.

And the best part is that it's not complicated, nor a dreary affair of counting calories, crunching kale, or suffering through special "biohacks" that will "lengthen your telomeres" or "inhibit mTOR signalling" or "upregulate your kajiggers". Restoring and optimising your health is a relatively simple and rewarding process. Once you pass the initial hump of habit changes, the fun begins. Trust me, waking up refreshed with an abundance of energy to focus on your ambitions while avoiding disease and degeneration is going to be a blast. All you need is someone to give you a roadmap. I'll also explain the reasoning behind my recommendations, as they may initially seem counterintuitive. This is not because I am a contrarian, but because you may have been misinformed.

In fact, as my understanding became more nuanced over the years, I have found much of the advice disseminated dogmatically in the mainstream to be useless or downright harmful. This is especially the case for older people who do not have the adaptive reserve required to bounce back from supposedly beneficial longevity practices that are actually doing nothing more than stressing and depleting their bodies.

It is my humble mission to remedy this and offer you solutions that consider our modern challenges, your busy lifestyle, and that you probably don't want to suffer through five-hundred pages of flowery bullshit stories and elaborate explanations of molecular mechanisms to uncover a few gems of applicable wisdom. By the end of this short first volume, you will have the knowledge and tools you need to make a meaningful impact on your life- and healthspan; future volumes will build on these foundations.

Will you live to 110 years by following the advice laid out here? Perhaps. It depends on how healthy you were to begin with and the age at which you started implementing the information. Since we're all battling entropy and the ravages of the modern world, there are no guarantees. I'm not even sure this iteration of our journey on Earth requires that many years. My view is that life is about the lessons we learn and the important work we do, not the chronological time we accrue. We should not allow our egos to turn it into a pathological competition of "who can live the longest".

But I am sure of this: If you implement the tools and strategies in this book series, the entire trajectory of your health will be transformed. You will have more energy to pursue your desires, to play with your grandkids, or to travel the world. You will sleep better, think clearly, and be calmer and more centred. Most importantly, you will maintain your physical and cognitive functions as the years go by. Does that sound like a sweet deal or what?

Before we begin discussing the practical aspects of longevity, I need to briefly introduce you to what I call the "primary drivers of ageing and dysfunction"—a.k.a. the things that are slowly killing you—because addressing these will be one of our primary directives.

Online Appendix and Longevity Program

I've created an online appendix with links to the supplements mentioned in the book. In addition, **if you are truly serious about optimising your health and longevity**, I invite you to request a free intro call with me to see if we're a good fit to work together to accelerate your progress. We'll do this using state-of-the-art functional lab testing and my health optimisation and longevity protocols that address nutrition, supplementation, gut health, detoxification, sleep, stress reduction, inflammation, oxidative stress, and other important areas.

Online Appendix:
https://HowToActuallyLiveLonger.com/vol-1

Longevity Program:
https://HowToActuallyLiveLonger.com/

Scan the QR code to visit the website:

---

1 Understand What's Killing You

Once I fully grasped the importance of proactively tending to my health—rather than waiting for something to go wrong before seeking help, as we have been taught to do—I immersed myself in functional and natural medicine. It soon became clear that the dominant medical paradigm exists primarily to extract profit by masking symptoms of disease with prescription chemicals without addressing the underlying causes, and the doctors were the unwitting henchmen perpetrating this travesty.

A microcosm of this was evident in my family. My grandparents got roped in during their fifties—you may know the worn-out spiel used to get the foot in the door: it either starts with blood-pressure or cholesterol-lowering drugs (or both) and before you know it, the person is on a cocktail of pills where each one treats a side-effect caused by another. Our society has normalised this merry-go-round of hell, but I resolved to *never* end up like that.

A natural progression of my research was to understand what actually causes disease and dysfunction, and thus premature ageing. This is where I think a lot of intellectual types get lost and confused. It is incredibly easy to fall down the rabbit hole of scouring studies to uncover minute details and mechanisms—much of which is beyond the understanding of us mere mortals—and completely lose the forest for the trees. At the end of such an endeavour, few of us would be better equipped to extend our life- or healthspan. For example, if you peruse the ageing literature, you will quickly stumble upon the "nine hallmarks of ageing", which are:

> ...genomic instability, telomere attrition, epigenetic alterations, loss of proteostasis, deregulated nutrient sensing, mitochondrial dysfunction, cellular senescence, stem cell exhaustion, and altered intercellular communication.[1]

Where would you even begin? Each of these topics is already so vast that you can specialise in a tiny aspect, earn your PhD, and enjoy an extensive career elucidating the various biochemical mechanisms at play. But for the regular person, it is infinitely more useful to understand some high-level concepts, then proceed to the practical aspects, because that is where the true value lies.

Now, I know I'm simplifying things *a lot*, but here is the part you need to grasp: The hallmarks of ageing pertain to **damage and dysfunction in our cells and their components**. That could be damage to the DNA in the cell nucleus or the mitochondria (the energy-producing organelles, which have their own separate genome), or a reduced ability to create enzymes and other proteins, or otherwise compromised defence and repair processes.

When you zoom in inside the body, **it is precisely this damage or dysfunction in the cells that is the true underlying cause of all disease**. If a cell cannot do its job properly or dies prematurely, it may injure its neighbours and cause them to malfunction. That group of cells is part of a larger tissue that may be part of an organ—for example, the liver or the brain. What started as an issue at the cellular level now grows to be dysfunction at the level of the organ, which is part of an organ system (e.g., gastrointestinal or nervous system). By this point (and often earlier), the organism—the person—can experience overt symptoms such as pain, fatigue, or debilitation. But it all started at the level of the cell.

How quickly this low-level cellular dysfunction manifests as noticeable health problems depends on various nutritional and lifestyle factors. Under normal conditions, cells can deal with the wear and tear caused by daily life. However, if they don't receive adequate fuel and nutrients required for repair and regeneration or the harmful factors are too overwhelming, the damage accumulates. The body will do its best to compensate for imbalances and maintain homeostasis for as long as possible—sometimes for decades. It does this either by breaking down parts of itself or by "downsizing" (i.e., shutting down functions). Over time, we may notice more wrinkles, age spots, loss of skin elasticity, or loss of bone and muscle mass, but these are preferable over serious diseases like dementia, cancer, or atherosclerosis (which is the build-up of plaque in our arteries that can increase our risk of heart attack, stroke, and a host of other problems).

Once all of this clicked for me, the path became clearer. I finally understood what it meant to be "proactive" about my health. I needed to figure out what causes damage to my cells, how to prevent or minimise it, and how to provide my cells with the nutrients and fuel they need to carry out their myriad functions. We'll review the major harmful factors next.

The primary drivers of ageing and dysfunction

Stress—that is what's killing you. It ages you prematurely and is a primary driver of disease. I say this without a touch of hyperbole. It's important that you understand I'm not only talking about the psychological stress most of us can easily sense—like trying to cook dinner with a screaming kid tugging at you or polishing a presentation the night before an important meeting. While our levels of this type of stress are sky high as a society, it's only a piece of the larger puzzle.

It is the *physiological* stress in our body, which can be caused by psychological or physical factors, that is incredibly pernicious. Not only are relatively few of us tuned into this type of stress, much of it cannot even be "sensed". We can only detect it with certain lab tests or when it accumulates to the point of causing noticeable symptoms or dysfunction in the body.

Since stress comes in many flavours, we will expand the discussion to include the major archetypal stressors in the body: **inflammation** and **oxidative stress**. I call them archetypal stressors because they can manifest due to a multitude of internal or external influences and can contribute to almost any dysfunction and disease you can think of.

For example, some researchers use the term "inflammageing" to describe ageing induced by chronic and persistent inflammation, which is also associated with poorer physical function and loss of muscle strength in older adults.[2-5] A quote from the literature summarises it succinctly:

> Chronic inflammation is one of the major contributors to age-associated diseases and aging and disrupts the normal functioning of tissues[6]

Oxidative stress is a state where our antioxidant and repair systems are overwhelmed by reactive oxygen species (ROS). The resulting damage may disrupt the functioning of our cells and their membranes and other components, including the mitochondria. And since a cell's ability to burn (or oxidise) glucose and fat for energy is a prerequisite for it to do most anything else, mitochondrial dysfunction can accelerate cognitive and physical decline, and lead to a lower quality of life. Oxidative damage in our brain cells can lead to neurodegeneration and premature loss of cognitive abilities.

> Oxidative stress (OxS) and mitochondrial dysfunction are implicated as causative factors for aging. Older adults (OAs) have an increased prevalence of elevated OxS, impaired mitochondrial fuel-oxidation (MFO), elevated inflammation, endothelial dysfunction, insulin resistance, cognitive decline, muscle weakness, and sarcopenia[7]

In simpler terms, unmitigated inflammation and oxidative stress speed up the ageing process because of the damage they inflict on our cells, tissues, and organs. This creates the predisposing environment for our two biggest killers to develop— cardiovascular disease and cancer. Because the body and mind are one, these pathological processes also underlie depression, cognitive decline, dementia, and other neuropsychiatric conditions.[8][9] No aspect of our body's functioning can escape the ravages.

Conversely, if you keep stress, inflammation, and oxidative stress as low as possible, you will stave off disease and degeneration because less cells will be damaged over the course of your life. It's that simple. These are *the* requirements for a long life- and healthspan. After that, you'll just have to watch out for any flying pianos and hope the sick-care industry doesn't sink its hooks into you.

Naturally, there are nuances we need to discuss. First, you need to learn which factors cause stress, inflammation, and oxidative stress. You're an adult, so I won't lie—the list is long. Damned long. We can thank the spoils of the modern world for that.

Figure 1 shows a simplified model of how some of these interact. As you can see, there is overlap between the areas; and factors often feed into one another in a non-linear fashion. For example, one way inflammation drives stress is due to the rise in the hormone cortisol (we'll discuss it in more depth shortly), which serves an anti-inflammatory role in the body. Toxins— whether metals, chemicals, or those produced by bacteria in the gut—are another stressor that drives inflammation and oxidative stress. My model is not comprehensive, as an overview is all you need. We won't get bogged down in details because, in my experience, making a few decisions can have a profoundly penetrating effect on a person's health.

For example, choosing to only purchase real food (i.e., no ultra-processed crap) that is ideally organically produced or wild-caught, will remove a plethora of pesticides, herbicides,

The Primary Drivers of Ageing and Dysfunction

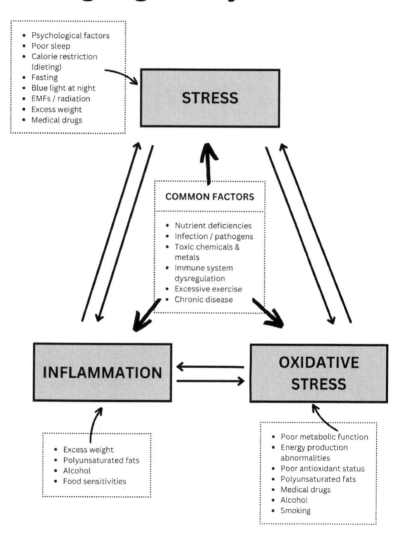

- Psychological factors
- Poor sleep
- Calorie restriction (dieting)
- Fasting
- Blue light at night
- EMFs / radiation
- Excess weight
- Medical drugs

STRESS

COMMON FACTORS

- Nutrient deficiencies
- Infection / pathogens
- Toxic chemicals & metals
- Immune system dysregulation
- Excessive exercise
- Chronic disease

INFLAMMATION

OXIDATIVE STRESS

- Excess weight
- Polyunsaturated fats
- Alcohol
- Food sensitivities

- Poor metabolic function
- Energy production abnormalities
- Poor antioxidant status
- Polyunsaturated fats
- Medical drugs
- Alcohol
- Smoking

hormones, emulsifiers, colours, flavours, and bugs out of your life. One decision, countless benefits. Less burden on your detoxification system, less damage to your intestines and liver, less "wasted" energy and nutrients to repair said damage, more bio-available vitamins and minerals, and so on. The list is pretty extensive.

So it is with dealing with the primary drivers of ageing and dysfunction. If you improve one factor, others follow suit. Less inflammation will result in less oxidative stress, which will result in less degeneration over the years. Improving your nutrient and antioxidant status will enhance your cells' defences against toxic insults and allow them to function well for longer—hence they will readily deal with oxidative stress and repair damage caused by inflammatory factors more effectively.

Stress Mode: Know it, Love it... Avoid it Like the Plague

I will be using the term *Stress Mode* to refer to the complex chemical cascade that your body initiates any time it perceives to be under any kind of threat. Stress mode is a literal lifesaver, but when chronically activated, it's a slow killer.

If you want a quick demonstration of Stress Mode, take ten breaths in and out through your mouth as quickly and deeply as you can. Don't do this while operating heavy machinery or if you have any health condition, and make sure you are sitting down. What do you notice? Your heart rate quickly increases and you may feel lightheaded. You may even feel a little "high". This is your *sympathetic*, or *fight-or-flight*, nervous system kicking in. This exercise might seem like nothing because after a minute or two, your heart rate will seem to normalise and all is well. But what you couldn't see was the surge of stress hormones (such as adrenaline) in your body; they are now elevated from their prior baseline levels. While your pulse may soon seem to return to what it was at the start, it will remain higher than baseline for at least several minutes.

The body activates the fight-or-flight nervous system in situations it perceives as "life-or-death". It causes your heart rate and blood pressure to increase and your blood vessels to constrict. Your limbs are mobilised for action while your digestion and other non-vital-for-survival functions are put on hold. The released stress hormones work to increase your blood sugar so you have energy to fight or flee, while also stimulating your fat cells to release fatty acids into the bloodstream.

Whether we're having an argument with someone in person or in our head, giving a speech to a large crowd, running a marathon, or fighting in a boxing match, the same hormones are released (in varying degrees, based on the intensity of the situation) to help us get through these activities—all of which are perceived as emergencies by the body. This is where Stress Mode becomes detrimental when chronically activated. Think about it: if all it takes is a few breaths to trigger a minor version of it, imagine how easy it is to be in this state throughout the day. Many of us are in Stress Mode for most of our waking lives. The worst part is that a release of stress hormones can exhilarate us, hence terms like the "runner's high" or "adrenaline junkie". The danger of this is that we may engage in harmful activities that we mistakenly perceive to be beneficial because we "feel good" while doing them.

You can think of stress as a spectrum that is different for each one of us. It's not activated with an on-off button—rather, your body turns it up or down with a dimmer switch. When you're well-fed and sleeping soundly, the dimmer is at its lowest. In situations like escaping from a grizzly bear or a cage fight, your dial will be turned up to the max. In between, you have all the permutations and intensities of stress. At a certain point on the dial, you enter Stress Mode. Figure 2 shows an example of where I perceive certain activities to be on my spectrum and which states and activities put me in Stress Mode. Naturally, it will be different in your case.

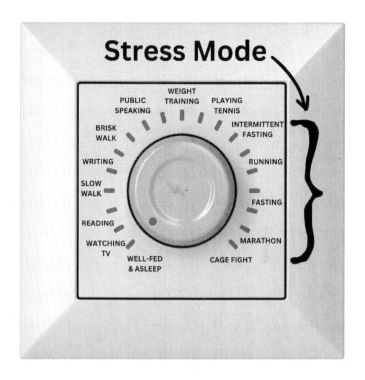

The goal is simple (though not always easy): you want to keep the dial low, and only turn it up into Stress Mode when you truly need it. You also need to avoid the delusion that certain activities or states are not stressful (i.e., harmful) just because you do not perceive them to be—this is critical to grasp and will be a central theme in this volume. If you need to sprint to catch the bus, complete a hard workout in the gym, or deal with an emergency, Stress Mode will be there to help get you through. The rest of the time, you need to stay out of it as much as possible because, as you will see shortly, the mechanisms via which stress hormones get us out of a jam are highly deleterious to our health.

Why is Stress Mode so harmful?

When you are in Stress Mode, your body prioritises the functions necessary for its basic survival. That means "nice to have" functions take a back seat. These can include physical systems and processes like digestion, but also aspects of the mind like higher thought, future planning, creativity, and joy. Now, you might think I'm exaggerating a tad when I state that stress can *literally*:

- Make you fat and give you diabetes.
- Cause you to get sick more often or to develop thrush or *Candida* overgrowth.
- Accelerate osteoporosis (bone loss) and sarcopenia (muscle loss and weakness).
- Precipitate cognitive decline and contribute to dementia.
- Make you depressed.
- Cause high blood-pressure and contribute to heart disease.
- In extreme cases, trigger psychosis.

I wish I was exaggerating, but it's even worse than that. The following quote encapsulates it well:

> Stress promotes adaptation, but prolonged stress leads over time to wear-and-tear on the body (allostatic load). Neural changes mirror the pattern seen in other body systems, that is, short-term adaptation vs. long-term damage. Allostatic load leads to impaired immunity, atherosclerosis, obesity, bone demineralisation, and atrophy of nerve cells in the brain. Many of these processes are seen in major depressive illness and may be expressed also in other chronic anxiety disorders.[10]

Furthermore, stress can send you to an early grave. A study that examined the link between levels of the stress hormone cortisol and incidence of death reported:

> High cortisol levels strongly predict cardiovascular death among persons both with and without preexisting cardiovascular disease. The specific link with cardiovascular mortality, and not other causes of mortality, suggests that high cortisol levels might be particularly damaging to the cardiovascular system.[11]

The important question to address is: *Why* is stress so damaging to the body? To do that, you need to understand the mechanisms via which hormones facilitate the stress response.

Cortisol's role in the body

We have all heard of cortisol, but few of us truly comprehend how destructive it can be. If you have ever felt anxious, irritable, wired but tired, or couldn't relax or sleep, your level of this steroid hormone was most certainly elevated and contributing to those states. Cortisol is produced in the outer region of our adrenal glands—the adrenal *cortex*, which is why it is also known as a *corticosteroid*—and is a member of the *glucocorticoid* family of hormones (a subdivision of corticosteroids).

The major role it plays in the body is to raise our blood sugar (or blood glucose) level when it drops too low. It is also released in response to other stresses, again to help us mobilise resources so we will have energy to overcome whatever challenge faces us. But *how* does it raise our blood sugar? This is the knowledge gap that we need to address.

As soon as your blood glucose level starts falling beyond a certain setpoint, your body initiates a cascade of stress hormones. Cortisol plays its part by stimulating the liver to break down its *glycogen* reserves (the storage form of glucose in the body) and release glucose into the bloodstream. At the same time, it signals cells to stop building new proteins and to increase the breakdown of muscle and fat to their constituent amino acids, and fatty acids and glycerol, respectively. The amino acids and glycerol are sent to the liver where they can be used to make glucose in a process called *gluconeogenesis*. Fatty acids are intended to be burned for energy, but this can cause problems in the body, as you will see later.

In this state, our muscles and fat cells become resistant to the hormone *insulin*, which you probably know is what signals to cells to uptake glucose. This is referred to as *peripheral insulin resistance* and is a nifty survival mechanism because when food is scarce, you want to prioritise glucose for the brain and central nervous system. After all, the last thing you'd want to do when starving is to go on a 5K fun run (unless you're living in our times, where doing fasted cardio is considered a viable way to stay in shape).

Remember, this is all done as a response to stress. In other words, the body is doing what it deems is necessary to ensure your survival, namely, to create energy that you can use to fight off or run away from the perceived threat. To that end, **it will sacrifice anything and everything that is not essential for basic survival**. Clearly, this is far from an optimal state to be in all the time. When in this Stress Mode, you are not just halting repair and regeneration processes while you're "dealing with the threat"; your precious lean tissue is being broken down so it can be turned into glucose—muscle, bone, organs, joints, skin, and even parts of the brain. This tells us two things: 1) Cortisol is profoundly destructive when chronically elevated, and 2) A steady supply of glucose is pretty damn important for the body.

Elevated cortisol is implicated in most health conditions

We know that cortisol levels rise as we age, but how do we know it to be a major cause of disease? The biggest clue is that it precedes and is elevated in almost every disease you can imagine. Beyond the more obvious psychological conditions like depression, PTSD (post-traumatic stress disorder), and addictions, cortisol is also high in diabetes, cancer, and neurodegenerative disease. It is even elevated in conditions you would not normally think have a stress component such as acne, eczema, and ulcers.

> Cancer is an example which clearly shows that high cortisol precedes diseases, as proven in experimental work on animals as well as in pre-disease epidemiological studies in humans.[12]

Logically, if cortisol causes disease, and stress elevates cortisol, it follows that **stress causes disease**. The solution, as simplistic as it may seem, is to keep cortisol low. And we do that by keeping psychological and physiological stress as low as possible. Not that this is anything groundbreaking—we've known stress hormones cause or exacerbate disease for decades. For example, below is a well-intentioned (but exceedingly naïve) statement from a paper that presented evidence to support the proposition, published in the 1990s:

> It appears that, for the first time, we would have not only new ways of treating diseases, but be able, also, to act to prevent them as soon as the 'high cortisol alert' or red flag indicates a build-up of cortisol which if unattended would lead to diseases, thus fulfilling the 'golden dream' of preventive medicine.[12]

How quaint. Too bad the "golden dream of preventive medicine" had its head bashed in a long time ago. Nothing personal, it's just bad for business. We're looking to get customers for life here, not lose them by doing silly things such as resolving their health problems, or worse, preventing them outright.

Don't be fooled that the sick-care industry doesn't know what causes disease. They know full well but are playing dumb. I am not talking about the doctors here, but the system which trained them when they were young and impressionable, and thus indoctrinated them into believing that diseases are mostly genetic in origin, and the only solutions are to mask symptoms with synthetic chemicals or perform expensive surgical procedures. And of course, they were taught that "natural remedies" are nonsense and quackery, and any beneficial effects felt are, at best, due to the placebo effect.

Today I realise that this system isn't broken—it was designed this way and is working impeccably well. For the incredulous, a quick glance at the current disease rates and the eye-watering profits drug companies are raking in provides sufficient evidence. In this profit-extraction paradigm, even the most well-intentioned conventional doctor is hamstrung, not only by their training, but by many other factors, including the "standard of care" and dependence on insurance reimbursement. If they deviate from the standard treatment protocols imposed on them, they may not get paid and can get in trouble and even lose their license. Thankfully, many doctors have seen the damage this has done to humanity and have turned to functional and natural medicine where they can be powerful facilitators in the healing process of their patients, instead of the unknowing accomplices of the morally bankrupt drug peddlers.

Having said that, it should not come as a surprise to you that cortisol-mimicking drugs are one of the principal tools of the sick-care industry. It is a perverse irony that they choose to "treat" illness with analogues of the chemical that directly causes disease in the body, but once you look deeper into it, this is on the more "benign" end of the spectrum of the travesties and crimes against humanity they have committed. (Lobotomy, anyone?) The reason I'm pulling on this thread is because the effects of these drugs show us an accelerated model of what stress—mediated by cortisol—can do to our health.

The damaging effects of long-term or excessive cortisol exposure

Glucocorticoid drugs (also called corticosteroids) are a large group of cortisol-like chemicals used to treat, or more accurately, to mask the symptoms of diseases where the immune system is overactive or otherwise dysregulated. Glucocorticoids are used in dozens of medical conditions, including gastrointestinal, skin, allergic, and autoimmune disorders. Their mechanism of action is to suppress the immune system—this is what makes cortisol an effective anti-inflammatory hormone in the body. But it comes at a price.

The short-term dampening of the immune response provides relief to the sufferer but leaves them more vulnerable to infection and fungal overgrowth. However, the longer-term dysfunction and degeneration caused by glucocorticoid drugs are the truly scary part. They are well-known in the medical community and are conveniently labelled as "side"-effects. Have a look at some of the more common ones in Table 1 and tell me if you know anyone experiencing them.

Table 1: Adverse effects of glucocorticoid drugs
• Weight gain and obesity
• High-blood sugar (hyperglycaemia)
• Dyslipidaemia (blood lipid irregularities)
• Insulin resistance
• High-blood pressure (hypertension)
• Increased cardiovascular disease risk
• Osteoporosis (bone loss)
• Muscle atrophy
• Myopathy (muscle pain, weakness)
• Infections and yeast overgrowth
• Eye disorders (e.g., glaucoma, cataracts)
• Anxiety
• Irritability
• Insomnia
• Depression
• Psychosis
• Menstrual disorders
• Skin disorders

- Hirsutism (unwanted hair growth)
- Swelling (edema) and fluid retention

If you're thinking, "Some of these side-effects are outright diseases!" you would be correct. What I found disturbing was how many full-blown conditions are recognised in the scientific literature as "induced" by glucocorticoids. See Table 2 for a list of some of them. Pretty staggering, isn't it? Let's briefly unpack a few of them.

Table 2: Steroid-induced conditions
A sample of recognised conditions induced by the use of corticosteroid/glucocorticoid drugs
- Steroid-induced diabetes - Steroid-induced psychosis - Steroid-induced panic disorder - Steroid-induced osteoporosis - Glucocorticoid-induced muscle atrophy - Glucocorticoid-induced hypertension (high blood pressure) - Steroid-induced cardiomyopathy (deterioration of the function of the heart muscle) - Steroid-induced glaucoma (eye diseases that lead to damage of the optic nerve) - Steroid-induced pancreatitis - Steroid-induced myopathy (disease of the muscle) - Corticosteroid-induced lipodystrophy

Below is a quote from a paper published in 1986, titled "Is atherosclerosis a complication of long-term corticosteroid treatment?":

...an increasing body of evidence suggests that prolonged corticosteroid therapy accelerates the development of atherosclerosis. An important element in this process may be the fact that corticosteroids induce or exacerbate several known coronary risk factors, including hypertension [high-blood pressure], hypercholesterolemia [high cholesterol], hypertriglyceridemia [high triglycerides], and impairment of glucose tolerance.[13]

The author concluded with:

> Any short-term clinical gains attributable to corticosteroid therapy may well be outweighed by the potential for accelerating atherosclerotic disease, particularly when treatment is initiated in younger patients.[13]

With drugs, of course, "short-term clinical gains" is all that is on offer. What is clear is that cortisol, whether naturally produced or a synthetic analogue, dysregulates blood lipids and blood glucose levels independently of what you eat. Another way to say it is: stress can raise your cholesterol and blood sugar. Hence, "steroid-induced diabetes" and "stress hyperglycaemia" are recognised conditions.

Now that you understand the mechanisms of how cortisol works, this may seem logical—it stimulates the liver to produce glucose and send it to the bloodstream, and causes fatty acids to be released into the bloodstream. These are the hallmarks of type-2 diabetes, which is rarely simply a problem of "eating too many carbohydrates", as the mainstream caricature of this condition would let on. In fact, it's well-known that glucocorticoid treatment can push a prediabetic person over the edge into full-blown diabetes. Makes me wonder how many cases of this condition are stress, rather than diet, related. The insane part is that when they decide to treat steroid-induced diabetes, they often use insulin, which has actions that directly oppose cortisol. That's like punching you in the head and then giving you an ice pack.

Now, since elevated cortisol results in sodium retention and potassium excretion, it is not surprising that glucocorticoid-induced hypertension, known as high blood-pressure, is a common side-effect of treatment. What that tells us is that if your blood-pressure is high, it may be due to stress, and not because you "eat too much salt"—another dumbed-down one-liner parroted in the mainstream media.

Think about this scenario: You have a morning appointment with your doctor, and you've skipped breakfast because you need to be fasted for the blood-draw. On the way to their office, your stress hormones elevate so your blood sugar doesn't fall to a dangerous level. You finally arrive at the clinic, where they measure your blood pressure and draw blood for the labs. Your doctor is concerned that your blood pressure was a little high; but this is to be expected, given your elevated stress hormones. When your lab work comes back, your doctor calls to inform you that the blood glucose level—which was raised by the action of stress hormones—is a little too high for comfort and enquires if you've been sneaking in too many cookies and soda lately. That must be it. Keep it up and you're getting a prescription, possibly a spanking too.

Can you see how ridiculous it is to draw conclusions and base decisions about your health—including doling out various chemicals with lists of side-effects longer than your arm—at a time when your stress hormones are elevated and skewing the lab values? Not to mention the "white coat syndrome"—a well-known phenomenon where a person's blood pressure increases due to the anxiety they experience when visiting their doctor. (If you think doctors would know better than that because of their extensive education, investigate who funded the medical education industry and whether they had any ties to chemical producing companies.)

What's next? Ah, what about steroid-induced cardiomyopathy (deterioration of the function of the heart muscle)? Isn't that clear evidence that prolonged stress can at least contribute to heart disease, if not cause it outright? And steroid-induced osteoporosis—cortisol inhibits bone formation, suppresses calcium absorption, and increases loss of calcium through the urine, which means that chronic stress, coupled with low intake of calcium, can greatly accelerate this skeletal disorder, which is the most common reason for broken bones in older persons.

Then we have corticosteroid-induced lipodystrophy, which is a fancy-sounding term for the movement of body fat away from the limbs and towards the face and torso. It is a remarkably common side-effect of glucocorticoid treatment and one of the most distressing to patients. An example is Cushing's syndrome, whose sufferers have thin limbs and a lot of stored fat on their face and around the belly and surrounding areas. This abdominal obesity occurs because while acute spikes in cortisol promote the breakdown of fat cells, chronically elevated cortisol stimulates fat deposition, especially around the trunk.

Unsurprisingly, complications of Cushing's syndrome include type-2 diabetes, high blood pressure, frequent infections, osteoporosis, sarcopenia (loss of muscle mass and strength), and various mood issues. That's okay though, we have blood-pressure lowering drugs, metformin, and statins, to "help" with all those problems. Oh, and for the anxiety, insomnia, or mood problems, we can always throw in some tranquillisers, sleeping pills, and anti-depressants. Trust the Science™.

To be clear, Cushing's syndrome is a condition of glucocorticoid excess—the cause of which can be drugs or, in rarer cases, a tumour that produces or causes the production of too much cortisol. While this is an example at the extreme end of the "stress spectrum", you can see how powerful the effects of just one hormone can be. (For a visual, search for images of people with Cushing's syndrome to see the characteristic "moon face" and abdominal obesity.)

What about glucocorticoids and mental issues? Along with depression, anxiety, irritability, and insomnia (which can worsen all the former), steroid-induced psychosis and steroid-induced panic disorder have been reported in the literature. One study that analysed the published case reports had this to say:

> We conclude that the cumulative data indicate that psychiatric complications of corticosteroid treatment are not rare and

range from clinically significant anxiety and insomnia, to severe mood and psychotic disorders, delirium and dementia. While tapering or discontinuation of the corticosteroid treatment may remedy these adverse side-effects, psychotropic medications are often required because of the medical necessity of the corticosteroid or the severity of the psychiatric symptom.[14]

Another example where more drugs are used to "manage" the negative effects of the initial treatment… Great business model they have going. I feel it's important to address the fact that there have been reports of steroid euphoria. This, along with mania and hypomania caused by glucocorticoids, demonstrates that stress hormones can give you a "buzz" or feelings of perceived elation. I believe many of us are not aware of how stressed we are precisely because of this phenomenon.

Another disturbing consequence of glucocorticoid treatment is steroid dementia syndrome. When it happens slowly over time, we call it "ageing", but when drugs cause it, we call it a "syndrome". One case report wrote about a 72-year-old man who, after taking a glucocorticoid for three months, "developed a psychosis followed by dementia". The author stated that:

> It was initially considered that the dementia was a separate neurodegenerative condition, probably of Alzheimer type, but when steroids were discontinued, he rapidly returned to his previous level of functioning. Reviewing the literature regarding the effects of steroids on cerebral function, the authors found that such cases of "reversible dementia" are not uncommon, although rarely given the emphasis they deserve.[15]

Terrifying, isn't it? You go to the doctor for help with your rheumatoid arthritis or other ailment, and a few months later you're psychotic and demented. Now you can probably understand why one of my primary longevity directives is to stay the hell away from the sick-care system, unless it is an emergency.

Finally, let's talk about whether stress can making you and me more dumber. I wish I were joking, but it's true. Animal experiments have shown that repeated stress causes atrophy of neurons (brain cells) in the hippocampus and prefrontal cortex of the brain. These regions play important roles in learning, memory, and executive function. At the same time, the amygdala, involved in the response to fear, appears to show growth.[10] Since we share a large part of our genome and physiology with other animals, we can reasonably assume chronic stress can have similar effects in humans—especially because elevated cortisol levels have been associated with poorer memory and/or hippocampal atrophy in healthy elderly individuals, as well as in patients with depression, Alzheimer's disease, and other conditions.[16]

Most cells in the body express the glucocorticoid receptor, which means that cortisol can interact with them and potentially signal them to dismantle. It may seem counterintuitive that the body would allow parts of an organ as critical as the brain to be broken down, but given its size and high energy demand, it becomes a liability in a survival situation. If you find yourself in a war or famine, all but your most vital survival functions will be given priority. These may seem like irrelevant examples because they are so extreme, but the truth is many of us are living in a "mini" state of war or famine for much of our lives (remember that Stress Mode is a spectrum). In order to live a long and healthy life, **you need to signal safety and abundance to your body**.

Conclusion

Fun fact: If you keep your cortisol low, you will look younger! Researchers have found that higher cortisol levels were associated with a higher perceived age.[17] Beyond the purely cosmetic benefits, higher perceived age has been associated with earlier death:

> Perceived age—which is widely used by clinicians as a general indication of a patient's health—is a robust biomarker of ageing that predicts survival among those aged ≥70 and correlates with important functional and molecular ageing phenotypes.[18]

In this latter study of 1826 twins, the bigger the difference in the perceived ages of the twins, the higher the likelihood that the older-looking twin would die first.[18] What that tells us is that if you keep stress low, you're likely to age more slowly, and if you "look" younger naturally, you're likely going to live longer because it indicates your overall state of health is in decent shape. I'll wrap up this discussion with a final quote:

> Psychosocial stress-especially when chronic, excessive, or occurring early in life-has been associated with accelerated aging and increased disease risk.[19]

I hope that was enough to convince you that the sooner you start aggressively reducing your psychological *and* physiological stressors, the better off you will be. Since I can mostly help with the physiological side of things, let's get right to it. Our first order of business is addressing one of the most insidious sources of inflammation and oxidative stress in the body.

2. Protect Yourself from PUFAs

My earliest memories are of grandma making her delicious *baklava* or *banitza* (a sweet or savoury traditional Bulgarian pastry made with grated pumpkin and sugar or feta cheese). She had a special technique to roll the baklava with a thin wooden rod that took a lot of extra effort, but the result was heavenly. I would hang around the kitchen sampling sugar, salt, butter, anything I could lay my curious little hands on. I still have vivid images of her drizzling sunflower oil on the dough or pastry sheets. We used that stuff in everything—from salads and side-dishes to frying meatballs and potatoes (of which I ate copious amounts as a kid).

Grandma ate little and skipped meals often; she always put herself last—so her nutritional status throughout her adult life was precarious at best. But I am convinced that apart from the sick-care system's poisons and butchery, Grandma's health problems stemmed largely from her intake of sunflower oil and all the toxic breakdown products that frying it creates. No one can blame her or my parents for not knowing the dangers to health posed by these oils. As the processed food industry's products permeated the food supply, our elders got the rug pulled out from under them. Who would have suspected a store-bought tomato or chicken would be so vastly different in quality from their garden-grown fare? No one thought the convenient replacements for home-made products—margarine, bread, salami, sausage—would be any different. Food was food. Few were aware of the importance of vitamins, minerals, or of the use of agricultural chemicals—especially the simple folks living in the villages in Bulgaria.

Decades later, many of us know better, but the damage has been done. Chronic disease statistics and the accelerating trends tell a story of woe. It is evident that most of the population still hasn't got the memo—that one of the most harmful aspects of the modern food supply is the ubiquitous use of seed oils. If we had to rank strategies for longevity in an order of priority, getting these slow poisons out of your diet, quickly and comprehensively, would be right at the top of the list.

Seed oils—a primary driver of disease

Seed oils, cleverly marketed as vegetable oils—who would ever suspect "vegetables" to be harmful?—include sunflower, soybean, corn, cottonseed, canola/rapeseed, and safflower oil, among others. You have almost certainly been exposed to propaganda portraying them as "heart healthy", but there is nothing healthy about them.

The main reason they are harmful is because of their high content of omega-6 *polyunsaturated fatty acids* (PUFAs—remember this acronym because I'll be using it a lot), which are extremely fragile and unstable, thus are easily damaged (oxidised) inside and outside of the body. These fatty acids get incorporated in your body's cells and tissues—"you are what you eat" in full effect. When PUFAs get oxidised, a process called *lipid peroxidation*, they cause damage to whatever they are in, or near to, which could be a brain cell membrane, blood vessel, or other important tissue. This leads to a chain reaction of damage that must be stopped by an antioxidant.

After understanding the dangers in 2018, my wife (who was still my girlfriend at the time) and I took drastic steps to remove seed oils from our diet. I didn't realise it at the time, but this prudent decision meant we also removed the very nutrients that protect those fragile PUFAs from getting oxidised and wreaking havoc in the body: the vitamin E family.

Ironically, it turns out that seeds, nuts, and seed oils are the best source of vitamin E. Since Nature doesn't make mistakes, there is a fascinating reason for this. Because polyunsaturated fats remain liquid at low temperatures, organisms that live in cold environments (e.g., Arctic fish, seals, whales) contain more of them to help them maintain their metabolic functions (saturated fats solidify at low temperatures, so PUFAs are in effect an "anti-freeze"). The reason seeds contain relatively high amounts of PUFAs is to allow them to survive the often-freezing winter months so they can germinate in the spring. The little bit of vitamin E in the seed protects the fragile fats from going rancid before the seed has broken through and set roots. Ingenious, indeed. But humans don't have to survive in cold climates without technological advancements, so our bodies need tiny amounts of PUFAs.

Here is the problem: Even if you completely stop eating all forms of PUFAs, your body retains all the ones you've stored over the last few years, which, for most of us, is a substantial amount. Your vitamin E levels will drop quickly, leaving these fragile fatty acids vulnerable to damage.

I was lucky that I caught my low vitamin E intake in 2018 because I was tracking my diet for a short period with an app called Cronometer. After some research, the (sub-optimal) decision I made at the time was to drink a shot of organic extra virgin olive oil (which contains vitamin E) with lunch. My wife found it quite repulsive, but as far as doing weird and gross things in the name of health go, that one was on the low end of the spectrum for me. Not that I kept it up for long anyway, given my distaste for olive oil.

Here is where our humble friend, supplemental vitamin E, comes into the picture. Whether you're still exposed to excessive PUFAs from your diet, or you recently got the memo of how detrimental they are for your health, you need to make sure you get plenty of vitamin E to protect the PUFAs you've stored in your body and have incorporated into your tissues.

Longevity tip: Protect yourself from the harmful effects of PUFAs with vitamin E

Add a high-quality, full-spectrum vitamin E supplement to your longevity program. Full-spectrum means a balanced mix of tocopherols and tocotrienols (there's four of each, for a total of eight). By "high-quality", I mean don't buy the cheapest supplement you can find. Look for a reputable brand that has the vitamin E extracted from a plant (e.g., palm or wheat-germ oil) and stay away from the synthetic form "alpha-tocopheryl acetate".

Ideally, you want to find a supplement that does not contain PUFAs, which are sometimes used to dissolve the viscous tocopherols. There are reputable brands that use a bit of sesame or soybean oil in their products, which is not optimal, but the antioxidant punch you get greatly outweighs the PUFA content of the capsule. I use those sometimes because the higher dose improves a person's vitamin E status quickly. My rationale is that most people who are just beginning to reduce their PUFA intake (or still have a lot of room for improvement) would benefit from the supplement even though it contains a couple hundred milligrams of a seed oil. At the same time, we could reduce dietary PUFAs by 10-50g or more, which makes a huge positive impact.

For someone whose PUFA intake has been low for a year or more, we can switch to a cleaner "maintenance" supplement that has lower vitamin E content per serving. You can see the online appendix (at HowToActuallyLiveLonger.com/vol-1) for links to the supplements I use in both scenarios and some tips on how to balance it with other fat-soluble vitamins such as D and K.

How to take: Take one capsule per day with a main meal that contains fat to help with absorption (hopefully not polyunsaturated fat). Most people can do this for one to three months to "top up" their vitamin E stores. After the initial period, and depending on the serving size of the supplement, you can take it two-to-three times per week and as you feel you need it. This largely depends on the quality of your diet—the more PUFAs you eat from processed products or restaurant and takeout food, the more vitamin E you'll want to take to offset some of the deleterious effects. But please keep in mind that vitamin E is not a magic bullet—PUFA reduction is *essential* for longevity, as you will see.

How long to take it for: It may surprise you to learn that PUFAs remain in the body for two-to-four years after ingestion. During this time, they are vulnerable to peroxidation and its knock-on effects. It is prudent to take vitamin E regularly during this time, even if you minimise your intake of seed oils and processed foods.

Why supplementing with vitamin E is critical to longevity

Seed oils go rancid easily, even when refrigerated—it is just a matter of time. Since they oxidise at low temperatures, you can bet they will do the same in your body, and even more so when exposed to the high temperatures of cooking.

The bad news, as already mentioned, is that when a PUFA that is part of a structure in your body (such as a brain cell membrane) oxidises, it doesn't do so in isolation. A chain reaction of radical formation occurs that needs to be stopped by an enzyme or antioxidant (such as vitamin C or E). The quicker our antioxidant defences neutralise damaging radicals, the less damage occurs to our lipid-containing structures. Vitamin E resides in various membranes in your cells, including those of the mitochondria (the "energy generators"), where it protects them from damage caused by "free radicals" or reactive oxygen species (ROS). Not the most glamourous job, but a critical one to do well if we want to slow down the ageing process.

Let's briefly discuss vitamin E's RDA (recommended dietary allowance) and people's intake and status, so you can see why it's so important to supplement with it in today's world. In the USA, for example, the RDA for adults is a laughable 15mg per day. Despite this paltry standard, the average consumption of vitamin E is only around 8-10mg per day—and I'll bet most of that comes from seed oils. Here is how they came up with the RDA:

> This value is derived from the amount needed to prevent peroxide-induced hemolysis [rupturing of red blood cells] in vitamin E-deficient subjects, which was determined from a limited number of studies performed and published in the 1950s and 1960s to occur at 12 μmol/L serum α-tocopherol[1]

Does "preventing peroxide-induced rupturing of red blood cells in vitamin E-deficient people" sound like this was intended to help you achieve optimal health and longevity? No, the RDAs were designed to prevent the plebs from keeling over while working the machines on the factory floor. The sad part is that most people are barely even meeting their RDAs, and those that do (and track it) are proud of it, as if they have done their job. We've got a lot more work to do, folks.

In the case of the vitamin E recommendation, I don't even think that doubling it would be sufficient in today's world, given the precipitous increase in our seed oil consumption since the 1960s. To illustrate, one review reported that in Americans, the subcutaneous (under the skin) fat's concentration of *linoleic acid*—the most abundant omega-6 polyunsaturated fatty acid—had increased from 9.1% in 1959 to 21.5% in 2008.[2] That is almost a two-and-a-half fold increase in 50 years. Did vitamin E intake rise in tandem? No, in fact, the estimates of the average American's consumption may be higher than what they are in reality, as a 2016 study put it:

> On the other hand, recent studies about vitamin E stability in vegetable oils suggest that the actual intakes might be even

lower than estimated. Commercial vegetable oils, which contain vitamin E, are commonly stored in the supermarket or kitchen in transparent polyethylene terephthalate (PET) bottles. Light, temperature, and oxygen availability have been shown to promote rancidity in these vegetable oils. Recent studies demonstrated that storing soybean oil in transparent bottles under household conditions might pose an increased risk for accelerated lipid oxidation[1]

The authors also stated:

> Therefore, the oxidative stability of vitamin E in edible oils is limited and vegetable oils might contribute less to vitamin E intake than has been thought so far.[1]

To put it bluntly, if you don't supplement your diet, you're screwed. A study published in 2015 termed vitamin E a "shortfall nutrient" because ">90% of American adults are not consuming recommended amounts of vitamin E."[3] The researchers also said:

> The prevalence of inadequate vitamin E levels is significantly higher among non-users of dietary supplements. With declining usage of vitamin E supplements, the population should be monitored for changes in vitamin E status and related health outcomes.[3]

If you have not already, now is a good time to accept that you need to supplement your diet in today's world. The sooner you remove any qualms about taking supplements because they "aren't natural" or "it is a little inconvenient" or "my routine will have to change slightly", the better off you will be. (I am not talking to you specifically, but to the other readers that may not yet understand the value of intelligent supplementation.) Remember that you do not live in the environment of two thousand, or even two hundred, years ago. There is nothing "natural" about the modern world—not the pollution, not the plastics, not the pesticides, nor the contaminated and deterio-rated food supply (most fruits and vegetables we buy resemble nothing you would find in the wild). Your nutrient needs are simultaneously higher (because of the extra burden on your detoxification system) and harder to meet (due to the nutrient-poor soils and food processing stripping nutrients out).

Why are PUFAs so bad for my health?

As I am sure you already know, there are various types of fats, such as saturated, monounsaturated (MUFA), and polyunsatu-rated (PUFA). To avoid turning this into a technical discussion, just understand that the more saturated a fatty acid is, the more protected it is against damage from "oxidants". Conversely, the more *un*saturated the fatty acid is, the more vulnerable it is to the lipid peroxidation process I mentioned earlier. This is be-cause more places exist on it (called "double bonds") that are susceptible to oxidation.

Omega-6 fatty acids found in seeds and their oils are more unsaturated (i.e., have more double bonds) than MUFAs (which have only one double bond, hence the name *mono*) like those in olive oil, which are more unsaturated than those found in co-conut oil (which is mostly saturated fat). Strikingly, the omega-3 fatty acids found in fish are even more unsaturated than the omega-6s, which makes them even more susceptible to lipid peroxidation (another reason supplementing with vitamin E is so essential).

It is imperative that you get a better understanding of the dangers of PUFAs because most people only see them as "not great" or as "empty calories". No. We are not talking about a benign dietary component that may simply increase your calo-ries and cause you to gain weight. We need to hammer home the point: these easily damaged and unstable fatty acids *become part of you*. The very cells that make up your body incorporate them into their membranes, including in your brain. That means your cells, you, are more vulnerable to damage, which, if allowed to occur, will cause you to age faster and develop disease sooner.

Below is an extremely condensed summary of why you need to avoid PUFAs not just "like the plague", but as if the plague got pinkeye from a rabid dog that was infected with canine-covid. The newest variant. On steroids. It's that important.

PUFAs are highly inflammatory

Polyunsaturated fatty acids like linoleic acid are precursors to *eicosanoids,* such as *prostaglandins, thromboxanes,* and *leukotrienes*—these are signalling molecules that can trigger various immune responses (e.g., inflammatory, allergic), increase blood pressure by constricting blood vessels, increase pain perception, cause the blood to clot, and other potentially pathological processes. In plain English, many of these molecules and their derivatives increase inflammation in the body, so the more PUFAs you have in your body, the more chances there are for inflammatory cascades to be initiated. More inflammation means more tissue damage and oxidative stress—thus accelerated ageing.

Looping cortisol back into the discussion, the less inflammation you have in your body, the less likely your adrenal glands will secrete extra cortisol to quell said inflammation. This is a prime example of how addressing one harmful factor in the body results in the reduction of other deleterious processes.

PUFAs suppress the immune system

It's not even controversial. For example, the first sentence of a 2007 study was: "*Dietary supplementation with polyunsaturated fatty acids (PUFAs) has immunosuppressive effects.*"[4]

Fun fact: Because PUFAs are such effective immunosuppressants, they were given to organ transplant patients in the past to prevent their bodies from rejecting the organs they received.[5]

We already touched on problems associated with a suppressed immune system in the previous chapter; another potential risk is that it leaves the body more vulnerable to cancer growth, which, probably not coincidently, has been associated with seed oil consumption.

PUFAs suppress your metabolism

It's well-known that farmers use corn and soybeans to fatten up their livestock. Knowing that, do you think the meteoric rise in obesity might have anything to do with our enormous increase in seed oil consumption? The two certainly seem connected. Research indicates that PUFAs can slow down the metabolism via their inhibitory actions on various aspects of thyroid hormone metabolism. As one author put it:

> Thyroid hormone, discussed above as the master metabolic regulator, is blocked at the production [58], transport [59], and cellular action [60] steps by PUFA. If fat, in the context of mammalian systems, is a storage fuel to be used during emergencies, PUFA is an agent by which that system is slowed for preservation over the course of the emergency.[6-9]

Thus, the hypothesis is that the release of PUFAs from our fat stores during starvation is an ingenious survival mechanism that slows down our metabolism to help us survive lean times. Great in a famine, but not so favourable if you want to stay optimally healthy.

Fun fact: PUFAs are so good at lowering the metabolism that some hibernating animals use them to get ready for their yearly slumber! Here is what researchers have to say about it (note: any bold emphasis you see in quotes is added):

> **Polyunsaturated fatty acids (PUFA) have strong effects on hibernation** and daily torpor. Increased dietary uptake of PUFA of the n-6 class [omega-6], particularly of Linoleic ac-

id (LA, C18:2 n-6) lengthens torpor bout duration and **enables animals to reach lower body temperatures (Tb) and metabolic rates.**[10]

In case you didn't know, some definitions of the word *torpor* include "a state of mental or physical inactivity", lethargy, sluggishness, dormancy, and so on. That is what a diet high in PUFAs will help you achieve—so if that's what you're after, tuck into those pistachios. Upon reflection, I don't think it's a coincidence that the rates of diagnosed hypothyroidism are the highest they've ever been.

Oxidation of PUFAs creates hundreds of toxic byproducts

The even worse news about PUFAs is they get degraded or oxidised into **hundreds** of toxic compounds (e.g., *aldehydes*), the most well-known of which are *malondialdehyde* (MDA) and 4-*hydroxynonenal* (HNE). Many of these compounds are carcinogenic (promote cancer) and genotoxic (damage the DNA), and it is no surprise that they are implicated in many diseases and ageing itself:

> Lipid peroxidation (LPO) product accumulation in human tissues is a major cause of tissular and cellular dysfunction that plays a major role in ageing and most age-related and oxidative stress-related diseases.[11]

Elevations in HNE have been reported in patients with major depression, bipolar disorder, and schizophrenia—once again highlighting that nutritional and lifestyle factors can contribute to more than just "physical" ailments. Researchers have found this toxic compound practically anywhere they've looked—from neurodegenerative conditions such as amyotrophic lateral sclerosis, Alzheimer's and Parkinson's disease, to atherosclerosis, diabetes, cancer, and even cataracts (an eye disorder).[11-13]

As I look back, I am certain the biggest contributor to my

grandma's atherosclerosis, neurological problems, eye problems (cataracts and glaucoma), and the neuropathy she suffered from in her last years was her decades of exposure to sunflower oil and its related toxic compounds, and the depletion of vitamin E they caused. Of course, her poor overall nutritional status played a key role, as that reduced her capacity to repair the accumulating damage. Maybe she would have been able to eat more had her gallbladder not been removed when she was younger—yet another travesty perpetrated on millions of people world-wide that can be avoided with simple lifestyle interventions. We will save that discussion for the next volume of this series.

Another PUFA metabolite, 20-HETE (20-hydroxyeicosatetraenoic), has been implicated in the development and progression of obesity, insulin resistance, and metabolic syndrome[14][15]—further evidence that these highly prevalent conditions are a product of much more than high carbohydrate intake in the population.

Keep in mind that these damaging compounds are formed even under "normal" physiological conditions. The body is constantly dealing with some level of lipid peroxidation byproducts, even in the healthiest of us. That said, what do you think happens when seed oils are heated to the high temperatures needed to cook our potato fries and other guilty pleasures? Trust me, you don't want to know. But let me tell you anyway: heating soybean or sunflower oil increases lipid peroxidation byproducts roughly by an order of a bazillion percent, times infinity, plus one thousand...squared. These toxins are then absorbed into your food. Remember that the next time you're at your favourite food joint.

> Continuous exposure of the oil to frying temperature (185°C) for up to 6 h gradually increased the formation of HNE and other polar lipophilic aldehydes. Additional investigations in this laboratory showed that HNE is absorbed into food fried in thermally oxidized oil in the same concentra-

tion as was found in the oil.[16]

Given that we build our cell membranes and cellular components with fatty acids, and oxidising a lipid causes a chain-
reaction of damage to those around it, isn't it quite logical that
these toxins are bound to wreak havoc on everything they
touch, including our brain cells, mitochondria, and anything in
between? I believe if we properly educate people about the
damage caused in their body every time they consume foods
cooked in seed oils, many would completely avoid them for the
rest of their lives. That's how bad this stuff is.

One study found that human subjects fed a diet containing
11.5% linoleic acid (mostly from sunflower oil) for four weeks
had significantly increased oxidative stress.[17] What more proof
do we need that this crap doesn't belong in our diet? The
amount of PUFAs they consumed was roughly 35g per day,
which you can get without breaking a sweat. For context, a
100g (3.5 oz) bag of tortilla chips can easily provide more than
20g of PUFAs. Throw in some mayo on your burger, a handful
of walnuts, and you're approaching 50g before afternoon tea.

Omega-6 PUFAs and heart disease

A question that may arise in your mind is: Aren't omega-6 unsaturated fats supposed to be heart-healthy? After all, we've
been getting clobbered over the head with this propaganda for
decades. Even now, the AHA (American Heart Association)
website is plastered with statements like "Polyunsaturated fats
can help reduce bad cholesterol levels in your blood, which can
lower your risk of heart disease and stroke," and "All fats provide 9 calories per gram. However, polyunsaturated fats can
have a positive effect on your health, when eaten in moderation. The "bad" fats — saturated fats and trans fats — can negatively affect your health."[18]

Yet, the fact that Procter & Gamble (P&G)—makers of
Crisco, a seed-oil based shortening originally introduced in

1911—sponsored the AHA in 1948 and catapulted it to prominence in the USA is nowhere to be found on the AHA and P&G websites or Wikipedia pages.[19] Go figure. Perhaps that's why bastions of "totally not horrible and paid-off-by-industry health advice" like the AHA, Harvard Publishing, and the WHO (World *Harm* Organisation) recommend you get between 5% and 10% of your daily calorie intake from omega-6 fats. And make sure you balance them with lots of omega-3s, because it's all about that the "ratios", you know. Of course, no mention of the potential harms I have covered here or the many others we don't have space to delve into.

Not only are omega-6 PUFAs, such as linoleic acid, *not* heart-healthy, they may actually be one of the primary causes of heart disease. If you search for "myocardial infarction" (the medical term for heart attack) on pubmed.org and narrow the search between the first record in 1916 to 1940, only 14 papers are returned. "Atherosclerosis" returns 12 studies for a similar period. For contrast, "diabetes" returns more than a thousand results up to 1940, and the earliest record is from 1788! Searching for "cancer" returns 2,612 papers up to 1940, with the earliest from 1783. Not to say heart disease didn't exist *at all* until the last century, but we'd have to be exceptionally naïve to believe it was common. The fact that it is now so difficult to find historical statistics by the year on our biggest killers is quite telling; we are supposed believe we will most likely succumb to cancer or heart disease and that's just the way it goes.

For a partial list of the evidence implicating omega-6-rich seed oils as a causative factor in atherosclerosis and coronary heart disease, please see Table 3 and follow the reference to read the full paper and see for yourself the mountain of evidence. It is beyond the scope of this book and way too technical and boring to go over it all. Just know that researchers have been questioning the "cholesterol and saturated fats cause heart disease" hypothesis since the very start in the 1950s, but their voices were drowned out by the narrative being trumpeted, backed by big bucks.

> Table 3: Evidence implicating omega-6-rich vegetable oils as a causative factor in atherosclerosis and [CAD] coronary heart disease (Partial list, for full list see[20])

- Linoleic acid is the most abundant fat found in atherosclerotic plaques, and this has been known since at least the 1960s.

- A meta-analysis of randomised controlled trials in humans found that when saturated fat plus trans-fat is replaced with omega-6 fat (high in linoleic acid), there is an increase in all-cause mortality, ischaemic heart disease mortality and cardiovascular mortality.

- Greater amounts of linoleic acid oxidation products are found in LDL [cholesterol] and plasma of patients with atherosclerosis.

- Greater amounts of linoleic acid oxidation products are found within atherosclerotic plaques and the degree of oxidation determines the severity of atherosclerosis.

- A diet higher in oleic acid or lower in linoleic acid decreases LDL susceptibility to oxidation.

- Linoleic acid is the most abundant fatty acid in LDL and is extremely vulnerable to oxidation being one of the very first fatty acids to oxidise.

- Linoleic acid metabolites promote cardiac arrhythmias, cell death, organ failure and cardiac arrest.

- Oxidation products of linoleic acid (including 9-HODE and 13-HODE) are found in infarcted tissue.

- Linoleic acid serum concentrations (as opposed to per cent of fatty acids) are higher in patients with CAD.

Seed Oils and Cancer

A paper published in 1996, titled "Diet and disease—the Israeli paradox: possible dangers of a high omega-6 polyunsaturated fatty acid diet" stated that despite Israel having "one of the highest dietary polyunsaturated/saturated fat ratios in the world", at the time being "about 8% higher than in the USA, and 10-12% higher than in most European countries", there was little to show for it in terms of public health. The researchers stated:

> Despite such national habits, there is paradoxically a high prevalence of cardiovascular diseases, hypertension, non-insulin-dependent diabetes mellitus and obesity - all diseases that are associated with hyperinsulinemia (HI) and insulin resistance (IR), and grouped together as the insulin resistance syndrome or syndrome X. There is also an increased cancer incidence and mortality rate, especially in women, compared with western countries.[21]

The authors of the paper wrote: "In fact, Israeli Jews may be regarded as a population-based dietary experiment of the effect of a high omega-6 PUFA diet, a diet that until recently was widely recommended." Ouch. It seems the experiment is not going well because cancer has now become the leading cause of death in Israel. A paper published in 2007, titled "Israeli 'cancer shift' over heart disease mortality may be led by greater risk in women with high intake of n-6 [omega-6] fatty acids", stated:

> Population studies of Israeli Jews, Arabs, and women support the association of high n-6 polyunsaturated fatty acid intake with increased cancer risk and higher female sensitivity. Research findings suggest that gender and sex hormones may influence n-6 polyunsaturated fatty acid metabolism and carcinogenesis.[22]

Evidence of increased cancer risk with high omega-6 PUFA diets started appearing as early as the 1970s. A well-known paper published in the Lancet in 1971 detailed an eight-year controlled clinical trial of a diet high in PUFA-rich seed oils and low in saturated fat and cholesterol in preventing complications of atherosclerosis. The 846 men were randomly assigned to either stay on their normal diet or to one where seed oils replaced the saturated fat. While the study found that fatal atherosclerotic events were more common in the group that stayed on their normal diet, the total amount of deaths were similar across both groups. The difference was the seed oil group had more deaths from cancer.[23] Not sure about you, but dying from cancer sounds less desirable to me than dying from atherosclerosis.

Since then, numerous studies have shown a strong correlation between seed oil consumption and cancer in humans.[24-29] Given the carcinogenic and genotoxic effects of the various breakdown products of oxidised PUFAs, I think you'll agree that it's best we err on the side of caution. I'll wrap up the discussion of the deleterious effects of PUFAs here because anyone that hasn't got the message by now probably does not want to get it. You know better, of course, so let's discuss strategies on how to keep them out of your body.

Long-term strategies

I sometimes tell my clients: *I don't mind if you go drink shots of Jaeger at your local club and sniff lines of coke off a dirty toilet seat, just please stay the hell away from PUFAs.* And I mean it. This is not the kind of matter we can slack on. You may have stopped using seed oils for cooking at home a long time ago, but it's possible that your intake is still too high. If you have the misfortune of eating processed, takeout, or restaurant food regularly, you need to double down on the vitamin E and think of ways to evade some of the oils that will invariably end up in your meals.

My current strategy when we eat out—which is rare because most restaurants use the cheapest and lowest-quality ingredients—is to ask the person serving us to tell the chef that my toddler is going to sample every single thing on our plates, and she has a severe allergy to seed oils. It works, and you ought to try it yourself—feel free to threaten lawsuits or grievous bodily harm if you think that is required to get the message across (just kidding—lawsuits are too time-consuming). Establishments cater well to people with allergies and intolerances, so if you ask politely, they usually oblige. Obviously, this will not work for the Colonel's deep-fried goodness—I hope that isn't something you'll be ordering too often—but it is relatively easy to cook a steak, fish, vegetables, or a stir-fry in butter or coconut oil, one of which they'd surely have. I would even prefer my food fried in olive oil than a seed oil, because the monounsaturated fats in the olive oil would peroxidise less. Better still, I avoid having to make that choice too often by not putting myself in that position.

Let me reiterate: processed, takeout, and restaurant food is not compatible with sustained health and longevity, and it is certainly not conducive to restoring your health if you have a chronic condition. I know it's not always easy, but where there's a will, there's a way. I advise my clients to bring organic home-cooked food to work, to purchase grass-fed or organic snacks online from reputable companies and stash them in the car and office, and to stick to basic foods when eating out (meat, fish, vegetables, fruit). As for those occasional times when you slip up—enjoy the meal, take your vitamin E when you get home, and think nothing of it. After all, it takes years for the damage caused by PUFAs to accumulate to the point of disease. One higher-PUFA meal here and there will not break you. Our daily habits exert the biggest impact, so let's focus our energy on them and not sweat the *occasional* indulgence.

To make sure you understand which fats and oils are high in PUFAs, Table 4 contains the list of oils to avoid as much as possible. And before you say it, I know—your favourite "X" oil that your favourite health influencer swears by is on the list. I'm sorry, I didn't make the rules (i.e., the PUFA composition of the oils). They were mistaken. Let's get over it like grown-ups. And no, it doesn't matter if it was cold-pressed or that you store it in the fridge—it belongs in the trash, or perhaps it can be repurposed as wood varnish or to fuel an old-school oil lamp.

TABLE 4: High-PUFA oils to avoid
• Canola
• Corn
• Cottonseed
• Flaxseed/linseed
• Grape seed
• Hemp seed
• Peanut
• Rice bran
• Safflower
• Sesame
• Soybean
• Sunflower
• Walnut

Keep in mind these oils are in a plethora of foods (e.g., mayonnaise, salad dressing, chips, pastries), so you need to remain vigilant. Also remember that since most chickens and pigs are fed a high-grain diet (even if organically raised), their fat is high in omega-6s—hence lard, fatty pork and chicken wings are not optimal for frequent consumption. You can, however, lower their PUFA content significantly. For example, you can trim the fat off bacon and ham. If you're cooking chicken soup, simply scoop out and discard the fat that accumulates on the surface (kudos to my wife for figuring this one out). I've also noticed that slow-cooking chicken in the oven retains the fat, whereas cooking it faster on a higher heat causes the fat to drip out. These easy adjustments make an enormous difference in the long term.

Remember, this is a solution to a modern problem; two-hundred years ago, chicken and pork fat would not have had such high levels of PUFAs because your great-grandpa couldn't drive to the store and buy a truckload of corn or specialised feed. While we are on the topic, if you search for "yellow grease"—the term for the collected used seed oils from restaurants—you will see that it is used as supplemental feed in conventional animal agriculture. If that doesn't turn your stomach, nothing will. How are *more* people not chronically ill? This is yet another reason to invest in organic and pasture-raised animal products (or wild-caught if you have the luxury) and try to avoid conventional agriculture if you can help it. The best fats and oils to use are:

- Butter (ideally organic/grass-fed)
- Coconut oil
- Ghee (clarified butter)
- Beef tallow

The "least bad" oils are:

- Avocado oil
- Extra virgin olive oil
- Macadamia nut oil
- Palm oil

Yes, you read that correctly. High-quality olive oil is a "least bad" fat to use. Not as bad as the seed oils, but it is not the answer to all your problems as certain health influencers would have you believe. I wouldn't go dousing myself in it and bathing every morsel of food in its glorious splendour, as it still contains 10-12% of PUFAs and is mostly monounsaturated fat, which is less stable than saturated. Using it sparingly is fine, but I'd stick with butter and coconut oil for most purposes, especially for cooking.

Why you may want to reduce your consumption of nuts and seeds

If the recommendations to reduce meat and saturated fat intake because they "cause disease" are bogus (and they are), and the advice to eat up to 10% of our diet in omega-6 fats is harmful, you can bet a *ton* of other nonsense espoused by the mainstream health press is bad for you. We will unpack more of it in the rest of the book, but let me explain why I consider keeping all kinds of seeds (cereals, grains, beans, lentils, nuts) out of our *regular* diet as an essential longevity practice. They are okay here and there in moderation, but should not be daily staples. And yes, I know epidemiological studies have associated increased nut consumption with better health outcomes and prominent health "gurus" speak highly of their magical benefits and the long-lived folks in the Blue Zones allegedly ate mostly lentils and nuts and plant-based blah blah. I couldn't give a rat's tiny hiney about all that—once you understand the types of compounds harboured in seeds, you see them from an entirely different perspective.

Seeds are the plants' progeny—they were not intended to be eaten, or if they were, they were meant to survive the digestive system intact and end up somewhere in a pile of manure so they could sprout into a new plant. To deter predators from devouring them, the plant concentrates toxins in its seeds. That's why you can't eat raw grains, beans, or lentils. Ancestral methods to inactivate the various toxic compounds include soaking, sprouting, and fermenting. Modern processed food companies largely eschew these processes because they add cost and time to the manufacturing process—yet another reason their products are so harmful. Cooking destroys some of the problematic compounds, but not all of them. Table 5 contains a list of well-known plant anti-nutrients, their sources, and some identified deleterious effects they have on health.

Table 5: Anti-nutrients in foods and their implications (adapted from[30])

Anti-nutrient	Food Sources	Health Implications
Lectins	Legumes, cereal	Altered gut function;

	grains, seeds, nuts, fruits, vegetables	inflammation
Oxalates	Spinach, Swiss chard, sorrel, beet greens, beet root, rhubarb, nuts, legumes, cereal grains, sweet pota-toes, potatoes	May inhibit calcium absorption; May increase calcium kidney stone for-mation
Phytate	Legumes, cereal grains, pseudocereals (amaranth, quinoa, millet), nuts, seeds	May inhibit absorp-tion of iron, zinc and calcium
Goitrogens	Brassica vegetables (kale, Brussels sprouts, cabbage, turnip greens, Chi-nese cabbage, brocco-li), millet, cassava	Hypothyroidism and/or goiter; Inhibit iodine uptake
Phytoestrogens	Soy and soy products, flaxseeds	Endocrine disruption; Increased risk of es-trogen-sensitive can-cers
Tannins	Tea, cocoa, grapes, berries, apples, stone fruits, nuts, beans, whole grains	Inhibit iron absorp-tion; Negatively impact iron stores

As you can see, beyond PUFAs, nuts and seeds may also con-tain lectins, oxalates, phytate, tannins, and even phytoestrogens in the case of soy and flaxseeds. You can't win either way: eat-ing them raw exposes you to anti-nutrients, while eating them roasted exposes you to oxidised polyunsaturated fats, despite some toxins having been inactivated or destroyed. Neither is optimal.

While long-lived peoples may have relied heavily on grains, legumes, and nuts for subsistence, this is something they did out of necessity, not because it would have been their first choice (and don't forget they went to great lengths to properly prepare them). When you have a dozen chickens, a couple of pigs, and a goat—like my other grandma had at her village before shops started popping up in the neighbourhood—you can't eat meat every day and are forced to rely more on plant foods. That doesn't mean eating more plants and less animal products is more conducive to longevity.

Again, I'm not saying you must exclude all nuts and seeds from your diet forevermore. If you truly like them, indulge occasionally. I just wouldn't rely on grains, legumes, and nuts for my protein (too low-quality and bioavailability), nor my carbohydrates (too much starch and indigestible fibre), nor my fats (too many PUFAs). I wouldn't rely on them for my vitamins (animal foods are infinitely better sources), nor my minerals (low bioavailability since many are bound to anti-nutrients). The one exception is organic white rice, because it is devoid of fibre, making it a cleaner source of carbohydrate.

When you understand the potential problems and weigh them against the purported benefits, seeds get relegated to the bottom of the food quality list, just above the ultra-processed crap. They are, and have always been, survival foods. If you can afford better quality fare, there is no reason to eat seeds, other than habit, preference, and lack of knowledge of the potential harm they can cause to your long-term health. I understand this comes as a shock to many folks and I wish it wasn't so because I used to love snacking on almonds, hazelnuts, and pistachios. And who doesn't like bread? But as adults, we need to do what is best for our longevity, even if we need to re-evaluate our beliefs about what is healthy and change our daily habits.

Finally, in case you have concerns about not getting enough essential fats on a low-PUFA diet, let me assure you that unless you get locked in a lab and consume fully synthesised fare, you will not become deficient in "essential fatty acids". Most foods contain PUFAs; even butter and coconut oil, which are predominantly saturated fats, contain 2% linoleic acid. Olive oil contains about 8% linoleic acid, while egg yolks contain 16%. I wouldn't worry about deficiency—I'd worry about the fact that we can't escape these fats! There are plenty of essential nutrients in the body that we only need in milligram quantities per day and that are extremely harmful in higher doses (e.g., iron, manganese, vitamin A). More is not always better and with PUFAs, more is certainly worse.

Conclusion

As you adopt the longevity-promoting low-PUFA lifestyle, you will gradually rebuild your whole body with more stable fatty acids. Though a slow process, it will make you more resilient to oxidative stress, which will abate the ageing process. You will also have less "inflammatory potential" simply because fewer of the precursors (e.g., linoleic acid) to inflammatory mediators will exist in your cells.

3. Evade Insulin Resistance (and Other Bad Stuff)

If you're like most of us, you've been unwittingly munching down on polyunsaturated fats (PUFAs) for the past few decades, which has caused you to accumulate a lot of them in your tissues. When we run fatty acid analysis with my clients, we sometimes see omega-6s as high as 40% on the first test, even in lean people. Hence, most of us have plenty of these pesky bastards stored, especially if we carry a few extra pounds.

Hopefully, you've taken (or have started taking) the important steps of removing (or at least minimising) PUFA intake from your diet and have added a full-spectrum vitamin E supplement to protect yourself. What's next? Should you just quickly lose a bunch of weight and get rid of those nasty PUFAs once and for all? Not so fast.

While the PUFAs stored in your body are certainly not benign, the last thing you want to do is start liberating large amounts of them from your fat cells. If you do—and especially if your liver health and antioxidant status are suboptimal—you're inviting inflammation and damage to occur in your organs, blood vessels, and other vital structures in your body. But there are other important reasons why you do not want to elevate the fatty acids circulating in your body. Let me explain why.

What is lipolysis?

The process of releasing fatty acids from your fat stores is called *lipolysis*. Each fat cell (*adipocyte*) contains many *triglycerides* (the newer term is *triacylglycerols*, but let's keep it simple), which is how we package fat for storage in the body. A triglyceride contains three fatty acids that are held together by a *glycerol* backbone. When fat cells are stimulated to release their fatty acids, they break down the triglycerides and send free fatty acids (FFAs) and glycerol to the bloodstream. The glycerol can be used to create glucose in the liver or to repackage FFAs back into triglycerides. The FFAs can be burned (oxidised) for energy, used to create signalling molecules (like the eicosanoids mentioned previously), or may be used as structural components in cell membranes or mitochondria. Unused or excess free fatty acids are formed into triglycerides that are stored in our fat cells.

There is always basal lipolysis going on in the body, and that is perfectly fine. Our heart and muscles prefer to burn fat at rest, and we don't want to interfere with that process. However, recent trends have promoted increasing lipolysis as beneficial, with notions like becoming a "fat-burner" or "metabolically flexible" being touted as healthful. In reality, they may be anything but—especially from the perspective of longevity and optimal health. In the next couple of chapters, you will learn why trying to "burn more fat" is not only misguided, it's likely to do you more harm than good. Let's lay the groundwork for your understanding with an overview of some nerdy concepts. Stick with me. I promise it will make more sense on the other side.

Why is too much lipolysis harmful?

To truly appreciate why we want to avoid being in a state of "elevated lipolysis" or "too much fat being released from our fat stores into the bloodstream", you need to understand that the process of lipolysis is largely regulated by hormones such as **cortisol, adrenaline, glucagon,** and **growth hormone**. Because these are **stress hormones**, it should be obvious that elevated lipolysis is a stress state. During starvation or an emergency, the liberation of fat to be used as energy is a wonderful survival mechanism. But the question is: Do you want to be in a state of stress chronically? A sane person would say *no*, yet it is staggering how many of us are doing the exact opposite.

Here is something most people don't know: **we can only burn a limited amount of fat at any given time**. Unlike carbohydrates, which we can process very efficiently if we're metabolically healthy (and lipolysis is limited), fatty acids we release from our stores that aren't used to create energy are stored back elsewhere in the body. It is estimated that we release twice the number of fatty acids that are actually oxidised, which means a lot of what we liberate goes right back into our fat cells after the liver repackages the FFAs into triglycerides.[1]

Given our limited capacity to process them, there is little point (and much detriment) in liberating more fatty acids from our stores than the body does during normal metabolism. In other words, whether we want to perform better, reverse chronic illness, lose weight, or just be healthy for a long time, **there is no need to try to burn more fat than our body would if left to its own devices**. One of the major ways too much circulating fat can be harmful is that **it will inhibit the efficient use of glucose for energy production**, and this can lead to a host of metabolic problems.

Insulin resistance and the Randle cycle

As you probably know, the pancreas secretes the hormone insulin in response to ingested food in order to stimulate our cells to uptake glucose. Its other important roles are (1) to inhibit the release of free fatty acids from our fat cells and (2) to suppress the production of glucose in the liver (the process called gluconeogenesis), as well as (3) to put the brakes on the breakdown of liver glycogen. This makes sense because there is no reason to release fat, break down glycogen, or make glucose if a meal just provided us with fuel to burn for energy.

Insulin resistance is a state where insulin loses its ability to stimulate glucose uptake into our muscle and fat cells, which results in a build-up of glucose in the blood. The other consequence of this state is that our fat cells do not get the signal to stop releasing fatty acids into circulation (i.e., insulin doesn't inhibit lipolysis as it should). While the multiple ways in which insulin resistance can develop are beyond the scope of this book, one of the chief pathways is simply **too much circulating fat**, the most common sources of which are having a lot of it stored in the body, a diet high in fat, or **chronic stress**.

The basic premise is this: glucose and fatty acids compete for their uptake into cells and burning for energy. If there are a lot of fatty acids circulating, cells will "reject" the glucose and it will build up in the bloodstream. It really can be as simple as that, at least at the outset. That's why obesity is associated with elevated levels of free fatty acids[2] and insulin resistance, and when an obese person loses weight, their insulin resistance usually improves. It's also why anti-lipolytic substances like niacin (vitamin B_3) and the drug acipimox (a derivative of vitamin B_3) have been shown to improve insulin sensitivity in lean, obese, and type-2 diabetic people. They do that by decreasing circulating free fatty acids levels, which allows glucose to be used more readily by the cells.[3][4]

We've known that glucose and fatty acids compete for uptake and oxidation since the 1960s; this process is called the glucose fatty-acid cycle, or the Randle cycle (named after Philip Randle, the man who proposed it).[5] Yet, the one-dimensional, kindergarten-level mainstream explanation of how insulin resistance develops is because we overeat carbohydrates, particularly sugar. We're greedy little piggies that munch on too many sweets and the pancreas cranks out so much insulin that our cells stop responding to the signal. They become "deaf" to it.

Or something scientific sounding to that effect. Right. Just like eating saturated fat and cholesterol causes heart disease because we found cholesterol in atherosclerotic plaques and eating saturated fat *can* increase cholesterol levels.

The insulin resistant state is pathological for multiple reasons. While the person is still relatively healthy, the pancreas will secrete more insulin to deal with the elevated blood glucose level. This will do the trick for a while—sometimes for decades. Most doctors are unlikely to catch this early as their routine screenings rarely include the fasting insulin marker (which, if high, is a big red flag). Your blood glucose may trend slightly higher over the years, but that's okay because they have an arbitrary cut-off, at which point they can diagnose you with type-2 diabetes. Until then, you're completely fine and don't you dare complain. Your cholesterol and triglycerides may be a bit high though—again based on arbitrary cut-offs that completely ignore your biochemical individuality and health status—so artificial lowering of those may be in order.

To make matters worse, excess release of free fatty acids not only makes your muscles insulin-resistant, it also increases insulin secretion and over time can impair the function of the insulin-secreting cells of the pancreas.[6] FFAs also inhibit the storage of glucose as glycogen—causing a further build-up of glucose in the blood—because if you are in an emergency state, it makes little sense to store glucose that you are going to need to run, jump, fight, or reconcile your spreadsheets for year-end accounts.

The free fatty acids activate inflammatory processes, which add extra stress in the body.[2] Because there's an excess of FFAs circulating, the liver takes the brunt of processing them; this involves repackaging them into triglycerides—many of which are stored in the liver. Over time, this can lead to non-alcoholic fatty liver disease (NAFLD), which, not-coincidently, afflicts 30% of people in the USA.[7]

Let me remind you that if a lot of the fatty acids in question are polyunsaturated, which is the case for most people, this process will be exacerbated. While the liver becomes "fatty", untold damage is inflicted to organs and the lining of blood vessels (which can contribute to atherosclerosis). To make matters worse, the kidneys respond to elevated insulin by retaining sodium, which can raise your blood pressure.

But not to worry, the sick-care system has your back. Your doctor will load you up with drugs to lower your blood-pressure, blood glucose, cholesterol, triglycerides, and perhaps a blood thinner to reduce chance of stroke. *Thanks, doc! I'll come back when all these poisons make me feel worse!*

As the metabolic derangement continues chronically, the liver can also become resistant to insulin.[2] This can further drive up the blood glucose level because the liver "thinks" it needs to make glucose through gluconeogenesis even though the diet is providing plenty. At this point, starting a low-carb or ketogenic diet may provide some relief to the person because it removes one source of glucose driving up the blood sugar level. However, it doesn't actually fix the metabolic issue, which for most people started as too much circulating fat.

As you can see, you want to avoid becoming insulin resistant if you want to stave off health problems and maintain longevity. And the primary fulcrum to leverage is to **limit excessive lipolysis in your body**. Like I said, this is a complex issue with many contributing factors, including PUFAs and their harmful metabolites, bacterial and environmental toxins, stress, and even poor sleep. We won't explore it in depth, but will nonetheless address its causes directly or indirectly.

There is another important reason why stimulating the release of too much fat can be detrimental.

Lipolysis releases stored toxins

One of the seldom talked about perks of modern living is that we all have toxic chemicals sequestered in our fatty tissues. This is not some woo-woo nonsense; it is a fact from which no-one is exempt—not you, not your shaman, nor the President.

These toxins, referred to as persistent organic pollutants (POPs), have an affinity for fat (they are *lipophilic*) and are resistant to degradation. Many of them were banned by the 1970s, but because they remained in the environment, they make it up the food chain by bio-accumulating in the fat tissue of animals. Since we are at the top of our food chain, we have the pleasure of being at the end of the line for these toxins. (Another important reason why food sources and quality must be one of your highest priorities.)

POPs are endocrine-disrupting chemicals (EDCs) that can induce inflammation, interfere with our thyroid function and sex hormone balance, damage brain cells and mitochondria, and impair immune and reproductive function. Because of their chemical structure, many of them are exceedingly difficult for the body to excrete. This is in part because a step in the detoxification process involves making compounds water-soluble, which makes getting them out of our system easier. Lipophilic compounds are difficult for the body to make water-soluble, so it seems like storing them in our fat cells is a reasonable strategy; if they were allowed to swim freely in our blood, they would quickly reach vital organs. The body understands the need to avoid this, especially considering the brain's high fat content.

> In general, once the lipophilic POPs enter the body, they are primarily stored in adipose [fat] tissue because of their lipophilic properties and then slowly released from adipose tissue to the circulation through lipolysis.[8]

So, if POPs are slowly released to the bloodstream through lipolysis, it stands to reason that we should not try to accelerate this process. If we do, we risk overwhelming our detoxication capacities and liver, which are already in a precarious state for many of us (as evidenced by the NAFLD rates in the population). That's why you *do not* want to do things that chronically elevate lipolysis above baseline levels. (If this was a drinking game where we took a shot every time I said "lipolysis", we'd be *wasted* by now.)

What causes elevations in lipolysis?

In a word, stress. Whether physical, psychological, or biochemical, anything that causes you stress results in a cascade of stress hormones. And the crucial part to understand is that, difficult to accept as it may be, many of the ostensibly healthy practices we engage in nowadays are keeping us in Stress Mode—thus causing chronic elevations in lipolysis. These include:

- Low-carb and ketogenic diets
- Intermittent fasting and skipping meals
- Calorie restriction (dieting)
- Excessive exercise (particularly endurance training)
- Prolonged water fasting

The mechanism through which the above activities trigger the stress system and stimulate lipolysis is through the most primordial of stressors to the body: depletion of liver glycogen stores and/or a drop in blood sugar.

Hypoglycaemia: the universal stressor

Our normal blood glucose level is between 70-100 mg/dL. A meal raises it and in the hours after, it returns to the normal for us level. The body is extremely sensitive to drops in blood sugar because too low of a drop will quickly result in us toppling over into a coma, with death following soon after.

Researchers have measured stress hormone secretion and hypoglycaemic symptoms to see how we are affected by a drop in blood sugar. When the blood glucose reaches 65-68 mg/dL, glucagon, adrenaline, noradrenaline, and growth hormone are already busy at work activating processes that will raise the level. At around 58 mg/dL, symptoms of anxiety, sweating, trem-

or, palpitations, and irritability are apparent. A further blood glucose drop to about 50 mg/dl brings about symptoms of *neuroglycopenia*, which is a shortage of glucose in the brain. Symptoms can be very disconcerting and include dizziness, tingling, blurred vision, difficulty thinking, and faintness. Deterioration in cognitive function is clearly noticeable at this stage.[9]

You can see that even before you experience the first symptoms of low blood glucose, your stress hormones have elevated. This is a survival mechanism that prevents incapacitating hypoglycaemia. If you have never had a hypoglycaemic episode, you may have seen someone who has. In severe cases, they may look drunk or extremely debilitated and may even faint. Less severe presentation may be of anger or irritability. (According to my wife, I was quite irritable and snappy during my intermittent fasting and low-carb phase. Not that there's any connection to what we're talking about here, I'm sure...)

It should be evident that maintaining your blood sugar level is crucial not just for basic survival but for proper physical functioning and certainly for excellent mental performance. If you let it yo-yo down multiple times per day, you risk metabolic complications that steer you away from optimal function. Research has clearly demonstrated that **after an acute hypoglycaemic episode, insulin resistance can occur as late as nine hours later and is mediated mainly by stress hormones.**[4][10] What does that mean in practical terms? For one, it shows that **any type of stress can contribute to insulin resistance and the detrimental metabolic derangements caused by it**.

To give you an idea of the scenario: You wake up and take your dog for a walk before breakfast. Your blood sugar drops within a few minutes. As stress hormones get released, lipolysis is upregulated, and the liver increases its glucose production. Your muscles become insulin resistant to prevent a secondary hypoglycaemic episode if they suck up all the glucose from the blood (this spares glucose for the brain and central nervous system).

What's interesting is that while most people will accept that hypoglycaemia is a stress state, many vehemently deny that skipping meals, fasting, dieting, and intense or prolonged exercise are harmful, even though the exact same hormone cascades are involved. In the scenario above, by the time you get home, you are well into Stress Mode whether you feel it or not. When you finally have your breakfast (or lunch), your body is much more likely to store the fuel you consume because it has been receiving signals of famine. It's not a big deal if it happens once in a while, but becomes dangerous when you do it chronically.

We tell ourselves cute fairy tales that even though we are stressing our bodies, it's beneficial because "what doesn't kill you only makes you stronger"—that's the hormetic effect, allegedly. Except the whole point of hormesis is to exert *minor* stress. Doing fasted workouts while on a low-carb diet, followed by sauna and a cold plunge is not hormetic—it's freaking stressful! The people who can endure that are usually still young and healthy. And while most of them don't realise it, this stress is not making them stronger. As their bodies adapt to the stress, they may experience gains in strength, leanness, or performance—but it *invariably* comes at the cost of their long-term health.

However, less extreme folks are often not that sensible either. They might not crush it in the gym while on keto but will work their asses off in the office, skip meals, run on coffee till lunch, let's not forget cocktails in the evening, then go to bed late, and wake up early to do it all again. Leading a lifestyle like this causes the same stress hormone cascades, albeit in perhaps lower intensity or with more breaks in between stressful bouts. But it still takes a toll. Then people wonder why they develop all sorts of health problems in their fifties, only to be told by their doctor nonsense like "it's genetic" or "you're just getting old". I'm not saying you shouldn't work hard, kick ass, and live your life to the fullest—I'm saying your life is probably stressful enough already without you trying to add further stress to it.

Conditions where lipolysis is elevated

How do we know increased lipolysis is not an optimal-for-health state and that we should not chase after it? Quite simple: lipolysis is elevated in stress and disease states. Here is an example: If we compare type-1 diabetes to starvation, we will find a lot of similarities. In the type-1 diabetic, the pancreas produces little to no insulin, which results in a build-up of glucose in the blood. If left untreated (with insulin), the body responds by increasing lipolysis and using fatty acids as fuel in most tissues. The liver increases its glucose output through gluconeogenesis and starts producing ketones at a higher rate so tissues that cannot use fatty acids have fuel to burn for energy. **These same exact metabolic changes happen in starvation**. The only difference is the type-1 diabetic's blood glucose level is high because their muscle and fat cells cannot uptake glucose from the bloodstream (as there is a lack of insulin).

Given that lipolysis is increased in obesity, metabolic syndrome, type-2 diabetes, and even cancer and HIV, I think it's safe to say it's undesirable to mimic the physiology of these conditions. If you have been led to believe that it is all okay and "you just need to adapt to fat-burning mode", I ask you: Why would you want to adapt to using what is clearly a backup emergency system? Why would you want to run on a system that works through increased stress hormones and the breaking down of your body? Especially when there is an alternative system that is not fuelled by stress. Because our favourite health influencers are doing it? I've certainly made that mistake in the past.

Whatever the reason, the fact remains that stress hormones age us faster and can cause disease to develop sooner. You saw in chapter one that "high cortisol levels strongly predict cardiovascular death among persons both with and without preexisting cardiovascular disease".[11] Researchers have also found that high adrenaline and noradrenaline (known as *catecholamines*) in older people were associated with a higher incidence of death or functional decline:

> …subjects with high baseline urinary excretion of epinephrine [adrenaline], norepinephrine [noradrenaline], or either catecholamine were at **higher risk for mortality and functional decline at 3 and 7 years**[12]

Their conclusion was:

> High urinary catecholamine excretion in high-functioning, community-dwelling older persons likely reflects subclinical sympathetic stimulation and is a marker of increased risk for functional decline and mortality.[12]

"Subclinical sympathetic stimulation" is another way to say increased Stress Mode without overt "symptoms" of being in a stress state. Just like having a subclinical (undiagnosed or not yet diagnosable) vitamin or mineral deficiency contributes to diminished longevity, having the fight-or-flight nervous system constantly "on in the background" does the same by wearing out your body.

In summary, you do not want to increase lipolysis above baseline levels too often because:

- It's a process driven by stress hormones—you're in Stress Mode (catabolic, breaking down, high-strung, fight-or-flight).
- Your body can only burn a limited amount of fat at any given time. Fatty acids that are not used get repackaged into triglycerides and stored.
- The increase in free fatty acids inhibits glucose metabolism, which can cause insulin resistance and its damaging consequences.
- The increase in circulating PUFAs can increase inflammation and damage to organs, blood vessels, and other vital tissues, as well as slow down the metabo-

lism.

- It releases stored toxins that can cause further damage and inflammation, particularly if they make it to the brain and other organs before we sequester them back in fatty tissue.
- High stress hormones are associated with premature death.

Pretty solid list of reasons, if I say so myself. Luckily, we have an easy way to block excess lipolysis from occurring (as long as we are not putting ourselves in highly stressful states).

Longevity tip: Use niacinamide to inhibit excess lipolysis and raise your NAD+ levels

Take 50-100mg of niacinamide two-to-three times per day to inhibit excess lipolysis. Couldn't be simpler. Niacinamide, also known as *nicotinamide* in scientific circles, is a form of vitamin B_3 that has an anti-lipolytic effect in the body. But here's the kicker: Niacinamide increases the level of *nicotinamide adenine dinucleotide* (NAD+) in your cells. You know what that means? Since ageing is accompanied by a gradual decline in tissue and cellular NAD+,[13] by using niacinamide to raise your levels, you're kind of a biohacker now. Congratulations. See you at the stem cell clinic. Jokes aside, the scientific community is pretty excited about molecules that can boost NAD+:

> This decline in NAD+ levels is linked causally to numerous ageing-associated diseases, including cognitive decline, cancer, metabolic disease, sarcopenia and frailty. Many of these ageing-associated diseases can be slowed down and even reversed by restoring NAD+ levels. Therefore, targeting NAD+ metabolism has emerged as a potential therapeutic approach to ameliorate ageing-related disease, and extend the human healthspan and lifespan.[13]

Sounds better than fasting and calorie restriction to increase longevity; I'll give them that. The primary function of NAD is to carry electrons from one reaction to another, which is an integral part of how we turn food into usable energy inside our cells. Without this energy, nothing can happen in the body. NAD+ and its related molecules (NADH, NADP+ and NADPH) are estimated to take part in over 60% of reactions in cellular metabolism.[14] They are the "central regulators of metabolism", and we use them for fuel oxidation and energy production, gluconeogenesis, ketogenesis, gene expression, DNA repair and regeneration, and many other processes. Pretty essential to life.

Niacinamide is a precursor to NAD+ and the best part is that it costs a fraction of the price of newer and fancier NAD+ precursors like NMN (nicotinamide mononucleotide) and NR (nicotinamide riboside). Using it also means you can skip the NAD injections and other expensive NAD-increasing anti-aging procedures that most of us cannot afford or don't have access to, or both. Buying it in powder form is even cheaper than the tablets, so if you don't mind the hassle of dissolving it in water or just directly swallowing it, you can buy the pure excipient-free stuff from many vendors around the world. The online appendix has links to the brand I use:

https:// HowToActuallyLiveLonger.com/vol-1

Another benefit of increasing your NAD+ levels is that the enzyme (11-beta HSD2) that converts cortisol to the biologically inert cortisone uses NAD+ as a cofactor. If the cofactor is missing, the enzyme cannot do its job, hence cortisol doesn't get inactivated—clearly something we want to avoid.

While we are on the topic of vitamin B_3, it is interesting to note that its *nicotinic acid* form, more well-known as niacin, is an effective lipid-lowering (i.e., cholesterol-lowering) agent that has been in use since the 1950s. Here is how a paper published in 1991 characterised it:

Nicotinic acid has had the longest period of successful use as an antihyperlipidemic and was the only drug that demonstrated a decrease in mortality in the Coronary Drug Trial after a 15-year follow-up (15, 22). Thus, nicotinic acid still holds a first-line position in the treatment of the most common types of hyperlipidemia [high blood lipids]. Nicotinic acid is especially useful in patients with severe hypertriglyceridemia [high triglycerides] (type-V hyperlipoproteinemia). It remains to be seen if lovastatin with its smaller once-a-day dosage and less side actions will replace nicotinic acid; lovastatin has been in use for only about six years[15]

And another from 1995:

"Niacin can be very effective and safe in lowering low-density lipoprotein [LDL] cholesterol and triglyceride levels and also in increasing high-density lipoprotein [HDL] cholesterol levels. In combination with other lipid-lowering drugs (eg, bile acid sequestrants), it has reduced the incidence of cardiovascular events and stopped the progression of coronary artery lesions. It may be the most cost-effective lipid-lowering agent currently available. At lower doses, sustained-release forms of niacin may also improve patient compliance.[16]

Here is what I'm getting at: At some point in your life, you may be told that your LDL (low-density lipoprotein) or total cholesterol levels are "high"—again, based on arbitrary cut-offs—and be offered a "lipid-lowering" agent (i.e., a statin) that you should take for life, lest your arteries clog up and you keel over from a heart attack or stroke. You should always follow your healthcare practitioner's advice, of course, but know that there are alternatives (such as niacin) to the "standard of care" that may have less horrible side-effects. My personal strategy is to avoid all that lipid-lowering baloney for several reasons, which I'll outline below. To start with, as a paper in the *World Journal of Cardiology* put it:

Often overlooked is the fact that numerous studies of cholesterol lowering have failed to demonstrate a mortality benefit and the benefits of statins may have been overstated.[17]

Not only is there no actual mechanistic causal evidence that cholesterol causes heart disease—the "large" body of "evidence" is mostly epidemiological data (read: statistical number massaging) and drug clinical trials (no conflict of interest there)—the lowering of cholesterol with statin drugs has not been shown to have a significant effect on reducing incidence of death. Furthermore, people with low cholesterol *also* develop heart disease:

> However, if one examines the original Framingham Heart Study data (as an example) it is clear that the cholesterol levels of those who developed CHD and those who did not overlap except when the total cholesterol level exceeded 380 mg/dL or was less than 150 mg/dL[17]

In the most influential heart disease study ever done—the Framingham Heart Study—the total cholesterol levels of the people who developed coronary heart disease were nearly identical to those that didn't, except when the levels were under 150 mg/dL or above 380 mg/dL (most of us have levels between 150-380 mg/dL). In other words, lots of people with low cholesterol also develop heart disease and lots of people with high cholesterol *don't*—hence this whole cholesterol spiel is a red herring. Here is what researchers who are not in the pockets of chemical producing companies have to say about lipid-lowering drugs' effectiveness:

> Since the introduction of statins to clinical medicine in 1987, several kinds of statins were reported to be effective in lowering LDL-C and also preventing CHD [coronary heart disease] events (mostly in 1990s). However, **unfair and unethical problems were associated with clinical trials reported by industry-supported scientists**, and new penal regulations on clinical trials came into effect in 2004 [4,5]. **After**

2004–2005, all clinical trials, performed by scientists relatively free of conflict of interest with pharmaceutical industries, reported that statins were effective in lowering LDL-C but no significant beneficial effects were observed for the prevention of CHD[18]

And:

Currently, the majority of scientists continue to claim that statins are effective in preventing CHD [coronary heart disease], but these claims are based on meta-analyses of reports, including those published before the EU regulation (mostly in 1990s).[18]

The above quotes are from a paper titled, "Statins stimulate atherosclerosis and heart failure: pharmacological mechanisms" where the authors state:

In contrast to the current belief that cholesterol reduction with statins decreases atherosclerosis, we present a perspective that **statins may be causative in coronary artery calcification and can function as mitochondrial toxins that impair muscle function in the heart and blood vessels** through the **depletion of coenzyme Q_{10}** and 'heme A', and thereby ATP generation. **Statins inhibit the synthesis of vitamin K_2,** the cofactor for matrix Gla-protein activation, which in turn protects arteries from calcification. Statins inhibit the biosynthesis of selenium containing proteins, one of which is glutathione peroxidase serving to suppress peroxidative stress. An impairment of selenoprotein biosynthesis may be a factor in congestive heart failure, reminiscent of the dilated cardiomyopathies seen with selenium deficiency. **Thus, the epidemic of heart failure and atherosclerosis that plagues the modern world may paradoxically be aggravated by the pervasive use of statin drugs**. We propose that current statin treatment guidelines be critically reevaluated.[18]

Good luck getting that "critically reevaluated"—we won't be

holding our breath—but it is encouraging to see that more academics are breaking out of the harmful paradigms in which they were indoctrinated. It's no small feat to "unbrainwash" yourself from the drug companies' massive influence on medicine and science, where fraudulent "research" from decades ago is paraded around as fact.

The important distinction is that niacin lowers lipids through more favourable mechanisms (i.e., improving some aspect of the metabolism), whereas a lipid-lowering agent like a statin blocks the enzyme HMG-CoA reductase, which plays a key role in cholesterol production, but also in coenzyme Q_{10} (CoQ_{10}) synthesis—a deficiency of which is highly detrimental to health and longevity. Not to mention the laundry list of other adverse effects the drugs have, which aren't surprising given that CoQ_{10} is integral to energy production.

It's obvious that the newer drugs were pushed onto doctors and thus on the population because "cost-effective" is not a viable strategy in a for-profit industry, and "safety" is barely an afterthought, given how many drugs have been taken off the market and the countless people who have died or been injured while using them. While it's true that higher doses of niacin can cause an uncomfortable skin flushing reaction, the fact remains that there are safer lipid-lowering strategies if, again, we even believe that the arbitrary cholesterol numbers we're told we are "supposed to have" are anything more than a ploy to sell a lot of drugs.

But here's the thing: blocking cholesterol production is a very dumb idea. Worse even, it's harmful. Lower cholesterol levels in people are associated with lower immune function, increased risk of infection, reduced antioxidant activity, and increased incidence of cancer.[19-21] Low levels have also been associated with cognitive decline. For example, one study found that:

Lower naturally occurring TC [total cholesterol, under 200 mg/dL] levels are associated with poorer performance on cognitive measures, which place high demands on abstract reasoning, attention/concentration, word fluency, and executive functioning.[22]

Cholesterol is critical to our normal functioning—it's a structural component of all our cell membranes, is the precursor to vitamin D and our steroid hormones (e.g., testosterone, progesterone), and is involved in countless other important functions. In fact, some researchers consider the plasma lipoproteins such as LDL to be a part of our immune system:

> Plasma lipoproteins (VLDL, LDL, Lp[a] and HDL) function primarily in lipid transport among tissues and organs. However, cumulative evidence suggests that lipoproteins may also prevent bacterial, viral and parasitic infections and are therefore a component of innate immunity.[23]

LDL has been shown to bind and inactivate bacterial toxins—known as endotoxin or LPS (lipopolysaccharide)—that cause strong inflammatory reactions in the body that contribute to many disease states.[24-28] Add to this the fact that higher cholesterol levels in older adults have been associated with reduced incidence of dementia,[29] and—this may surprise you—lower mortality (i.e., reduced incidence of death).[30]

> The impact of total serum cholesterol as a risk factor for cardiovascular disease decreases with age, which casts doubt on the necessity for cholesterol-lowering therapy in the elderly.[30]

The authors of the paper cited above also stated this:

> In people older than 85 years, high total cholesterol concentrations are associated with longevity owing to lower mortality from cancer and infection.[30]

How can something that is so "deadly" in middle age become

less of a risk factor as we grow older? What sort of rationalisations must we go through to accept such nonsensical notions? Truly harmful factors—nutrient deficiencies, toxins, pathogens, radiation—certainly do not become less detrimental as you reach your golden years. Yet, research has repeatedly found that lower cholesterol levels are associated with higher all-cause mortality in older adults.[31][32] Could it be...that we got scammed, big time? Knowing the track-record of the companies involved and having delved deeper into the matter, I've made up my mind. I'll let you decide for yourself.

Plenty of other authors have dealt with this topic in great detail, so I'll wrap up with this: A "desirable" total cholesterol level is considered to be under 200 mg/dL by the mainstream medical establishment. This nice and round number was basically sucked out of someone's thumb. Based on all-cause mortality data for 2002 from the WHO Mortality Database and mean total cholesterol data (in men, 2005) from the British Heart Foundation statistics—from 164 countries—there appears to be a "sweet spot" of 200 to 240 mg/dL, where all-cause mortality is lowest.

In other words, I personally would not worry one bit if my cholesterol was in this range—in fact, if it was less than 200 mg/dL, I'd be somewhat concerned. And I would never allow myself to be manipulated and scared into taking an unnecessary lipid-lowering chemical. Luckily, I would never go to a conventional doctor unless it's an emergency, so I won't have to have that awkward conversation. It's worth educating oneself about the risks and benefits of all interventions, and I have learned that—for me—most conventional interventions are likely to cause more harm than the often-imaginary problems they purport to solve. With cholesterol, this "lower is better" pseudoscientific propaganda has caused untold damage to the last couple of generations, and it does not seem to be slowing down.

Let me be clear about this: *truly* high cholesterol does indicate a metabolic problem, but the solution is not to lower the levels artificially and chase specific numbers on a lipid panel.

That is so preposterous that it's almost funny how it is all the "pinnacle" of modern medicine has to offer—with the brightest minds and trillions of dollars having been spent on all the research and advancements. (Of course, it is not funny because hundreds of millions of people have and are still suffering at the hands of this criminal behaviour.) The *actual* solution is to figure out what metabolic issue is causing the high numbers, address it, and let the cholesterol levels go to where your body deems is appropriate—which will vary through the different stages of your life.

It's quite relevant to this discussion to know that low thyroid function is a common cause of high cholesterol.[33][34] And here is where what we've covered in this chapter ties together. Niacinamide can help you inhibit excess lipolysis and enhance energy metabolism, which will support your health and longevity goals, but it will not work miracles if you are engaging in stressful "lipolytic" activities such as excessive physical exertion, calorie restriction and various forms of fasting or low-carbohydrate diets. Not only are these going to increase lipolysis and stress in your body, but they are also likely to lower your thyroid function and thus lower your metabolic rate. This may raise your cholesterol, but more importantly, can cause various health issues to manifest.

Not coincidently, older people with higher active thyroid hormone (T3) have higher muscle mass and better physical performance.[35][36] And since we know decreased muscle mass and strength are reliable early mortality predictors, keeping our thyroid functioning well into old age should be among our top priorities.

This directly opposes what some longevity "experts" espouse—that we must keep our metabolism low because we will wear ourselves out faster, as if we are a simple machine and not a complex, adaptive, and self-regenerating miracle of Nature. The century-old "rate of living" *theory* that feeds this religious belief (yes, very scientific) is completely debunked by the fact that birds and bats—creatures with high metabolisms—live long lives (e.g., some macaws can live to more than a hundred years).

Conclusion

To prevent insulin resistance, excess lipolysis, a lowered metabolism, and all their deleterious consequences, you need to avoid sending chronic signals of war and famine to your body. The good news is that it's relatively easy to signal safety and abundance. For many of us, it simply means stopping the ostensibly healthy, but in reality, counterproductive, practices we've adopted.

4. Signal Abundance to Your Body — Part 1

They may send me to the guillotine for this heresy, but you need to understand that **low-carbohydrate and ketogenic diets are _not_ compatible with longevity**. In my work with clients, I see the damage the low-carb movement has done, so I feel it's imperative that we educate more people about the potential harm. It is subtle in that early-on we can only really catch issues with lab testing, but the ramifications are long term and can be difficult to reverse.

It's quite distressing to see how carb-phobic we've become as a society. I see folks skipping carbohydrates at dinner because they are afraid they will get stored as fat or because they think they "don't need energy" while they sleep. Never mind the fact that only about 30% of our daily energy expenditure contributes to physical activity—the brain, liver, kidneys, and heart consume a whopping 60% of the energy we produce!

I also see others who say they "went keto" because they were led to believe it's a miracle weight-loss tool or the key to optimising their physical and mental performance, after which they tell me their main health complaints are weight gain and brain fog or issues related to hormone imbalance... And we need to figure what the "culprit" is... Perhaps it is parasites, or heavy metals, or mould toxicity. And while often there _are_ underlying imbalances that we discover with lab testing, the anti-carb propaganda has caused many of us to become deficient in the most fundamental requisite for life—energy.

Hence, I hope to warn you that *clean* carbohydrates (*not* crappy glyphosate-laden cereals, grains, or breads) are not the Devil, and ample amounts of them should be part of our diet if we want to thrive (not just survive) for a long time. I recommend familiarising yourself with the rationale presented in this chapter even if you are not on a low-carb diet or ketogenic diet, lest some sweet-talking devil seduce you into trying them. There is also a fair chance you are not eating an optimal amount of carbohydrates (most of my female clients usually aren't when we begin working together) and increasing them could improve your energy levels, sleep, mood, libido, and mental performance.

Longevity tip: Ditch the low-carb/keto diet

When I got onto the ketogenic diet in 2018, it felt as if I had discovered the Holy Grail. I was slamming back Bulletproof coffees with C8 MCT oil and butter like hotcakes. My love of meat and all animal foods ensured my excursions into Paleo, low-carb, and carnivore were most pleasurable, so please understand I am not "anti-" meat or fat or anything like that. This is about the mechanisms via which the body operates while on a diet low in carbohydrates. I believe if more of us understood *how* it all worked, many would be dissuaded from these diets to the betterment of their long-term health.

Let me briefly share my experience with low-carb diets.

After a gruelling 2016 of intense preparation for my first-ever Muay Thai fight (whilst on a fully plant-based diet) that I needed to cross off my bucket list, I had spent 2017 working full-time, attending college in the evenings and on weekends, and pursuing various other certifications. I was doing plenty of cycling and walking in going to all these places, but my busy schedule prevented me from cooking at home, which meant I was eating processed and prepared food daily. Naturally, this caused me to gain a few extra pounds.

Then the Lord shined his light down upon me. I started listening to some biohacker podcasts in 2018 and it was all *"low-carb is the best thing since sliced cheese"* and *"keto will cure what ails ya"*. Ketones will solve world hunger. Our ancestors did it, so it is totally the most optimalest thing you must do if you want to live to five score and eleventy years. And boy did dumb ole Christian eat it up like the plant-based diet two years prior.

Just like winning the first time you play poker or slots can turn you into a dragon-chasing gambling addict, losing weight quickly at the start of a new eating regimen can warp your perception of how good-for-you it actually is. Your initial success with a diet is all about context. If you are on the standard Western fare of glorified slop and toxic seed oils, transitioning to almost any diet will help you feel better and improve your health. It doesn't matter if it is vegan, carnivore, Paleo, gluten-free, or keto/low-carb. The key is becoming more intentional about what you put in your body and eschewing the junk.

As an example, in 2016, I lost close to 10kg (22lbs) in three months when I transitioned to eating fully plant-based. The weight loss occurred because I removed a ton of processed crap and started cooking most meals at home—not necessarily because eating a bunch of fart-inducing beans, lentils, and garbage grains was so healthy (the intense martial arts training schedule also helped).

So it was with my foray into the low-carb and keto world. After the "less-than-optimal" dietary period, I started focusing heavily on food quality: certified organic, pastured, wild-caught, blessed by a holy man, that sort of thing. And what do you know, a few months later I was being complimented that the weight was "melting" off me. Life was good. All hail butter!

However, none of this meant that a diet low in carbohydrates was in any way optimal for longevity, or even for decent health in the intermediate term. I was running more blood work back then, and the signs were there—I just didn't have the nuanced understanding to spot them. My TSH (thyroid stimulating hormone) was creeping up over the months, which was an indication that my metabolism was slowing. My cholesterol was also steadily rising—it hit 300 mg/dL at one point, which would make your conventional doctor's eyes bleed. The story I told myself was along the lines of: *"Of course my cholesterol is high, I'm eating lots of saturated fat. Everything is fine. The whole 'cholesterol causes heart disease' narrative is lies and propaganda designed to sell you cholesterol-lowering drugs."* And while that latter part is true, as I explained in the previous chapter, too high of a cholesterol level *does* indicate that there is an underlying issue.

Luckily for me, sort of, I abandoned the keto diet to experiment with the Paleo and carnivore diets, including a period of eating raw meat and organs. That was fun for a while until I got parasites, most likely from some uncooked meat. Overall, it was a rich learning experience. The journey was a necessary part of earning my stripes as a health practitioner; I made a lot of mistakes that my readers and clients won't have to make, though if they do, we'll be able to reverse the damage faster.

The game changer for me was discovering the work of William Wollcott, PhD and his book, *The Metabolic Typing Diet*. Briefly, using the Metabolic Typing resources, you figure out your own type and what ranges of macronutrients would work best for you, then you experiment to zero-in on the right ratios for you. What was interesting is that my metabolic type was the "low-carb" type in Wollcott's model, but even then they recommend about 30% of the calories to come from carbohydrate, which is a moderate amount. I felt exceptionally well on that diet. I was still eating plenty of my favourite meat, butter, and other animal products, but the increase in carbohydrates helped me to stay full for longer and avoid the sweet cravings after a meal of only protein and fat (which, in hindsight was a massive clue that I needed to eat some carbs).

Later, after discovering the work of Raymond Peat, PhD and experimenting with really high carb consumption, clean carbohydrates (e.g., honey, fruit, white rice) were completely vindicated in my book. This was a liberating experience, like the enjoyment of eating a steak without worrying that it was going to give me cancer or heart disease (remnants of the brainwashing from my plant-based phase that deeper research had undone). As it turns out, craving sweet food is natural. It is an instinct. The mainstream narrative tries to condition us to fight it, but the fact remains that we have a blood *glucose* level and, as you as saw earlier, the body will go to great lengths to maintain it, including sacrificing your muscles, bones, and organs. To restrict the fuel that is most preferred by the body (and especially the brain) is pure madness.

Why low-carb and ketogenic diets are not optimal for long-term health

Let's start with the ketogenic diet. The reason it is not optimal for longevity is because it **mimics starvation**. It was designed specifically for that purpose. Go on pubmed.org and you will see peer-reviewed papers refer to it that way. And it wasn't even intended to be used long-term for the purpose it was created, which was to help children with hard-to-control epilepsy. Now, this is a rhetorical question: Do you think signalling to your body for weeks or months at a time that it's in a state of famine is going to be beneficial or detrimental to your health? Exactly.

Let's look at what happens to your body when you start a ketogenic diet. During the first couple of days, you are still running predominantly on glucose as your liver and muscle glycogen are gradually depleted. As this happens, stress hormones such as glucagon, cortisol, and adrenaline start increasing the breakdown of fats into free fatty acids (lipolysis) and stimulating the liver to crank out glucose via gluconeogenesis. The substrates for glucose production include the glycerol backbone from the broken-down triglycerides, as well as protein from your diet and whatever muscle, organ, and other lean tissue gets broken down (of which there will be plenty, because you need to keep protein intake low-to-moderate in order to enter the ketogenic state).

Eventually, the liver starts producing ketones from fatty acids, which can be burned (oxidised) for energy by the brain and other tissues. This miraculous survival mechanism allowed our fore-bearers to endure extreme hardships so that today we can vegetate on the couch watching Netflix and posting snide comments under YouTube videos. Thanks, y'all.

Getting into ketosis does provide relief in terms of how much lean tissue gets broken down to support gluconeogenesis, but it will never completely alleviate that stress because certain cells—the ones that have few or no mitochondria—can only run on glucose. Examples of cells with no mitochondria include the red blood cells and those in our eyes (cornea, lens, and retina), while cells with few mitochondria include parts of the kidney, certain white blood cells, and those in the testes. (As an aside, I wonder if the recent popularity of ketogenic and low-carb diets is contributing to the plummeting male fertility we are now witnessing... During long-term glucose deprivation, the brain, nervous system, kidneys, and blood cells would most definitely take priority over "nice-to-haves" like testicular health and being fertile, given they are not critical to immediate survival.)

Low-carb diet proponents may say that the process of gluconeogenesis will swiftly make up for any glucose deficit in the body. It is true that the liver can make plenty of glucose, but we must never forget that **this process is driven by stress hormones**. The result is lean tissue getting broken down and an increase in lipolysis (not something we want to increase).

The next argument may be that our dietary protein will provide plenty of substrates from which to produce glucose, so the body will spare our muscles and there is absolutely nothing to worry about. However, as one paper singing praises for the keto diet put it:

Casein and meat protein can be converted to glucose at about 50% efficiency, so approximately 100 g of protein can produce 50 g of glucose via gluconeogenesis.[1]

Wow. Are you freaking kidding me? They just glossed over that like it was nothing. A kilogram (2.2 lbs) of organic beef costs about $50 in my neck of the woods. Are you telling me that on a keto diet, a bunch of that delicious and expensive steak is going to be wasted just to get converted to glucose? A kilogram of honey costs less than fifteen bucks and provides 800g of clean carbohydrates. It pains me to think how much high-quality meat I wasted by turning it into glucose during my low-carb days…

Which brings me to the question: If a significant portion of the protein you eat on a keto diet gets converted to glucose, and eating too much protein will kick you out of ketosis, how are we supposed to get enough protein to build and repair tissue and synthesise the thousands of enzymes, hormones, neurotransmitters, and other vital proteins we need to *thrive* (not just survive)? It seems like glucose is pretty damn important to the body if it will sacrifice quality protein to produce it. I don't see how this can be an optimal diet for maintaining muscle mass as we age, much less building more of it.

Another argument for the keto diet is that we can produce plenty of glucose from the breakdown of triglycerides—the three fatty acids are burned for energy or converted to ketones, and the glycerol backbone that held them together can travel to the liver to be converted to glucose. Sounds great on paper, but 1000g of triglycerides would only allow for 100g of glucose to be created (it takes two glycerol molecules to make one molecule of glucose). That is about six tablespoons of honey. Let's simplify the math and assume 1g of triglycerides is around 9 kcal; even if you consume 3000 kcal of fat in a day—a whopping 333 grams of it—you'll only make about 33g of glucose. In short, this is a negligible pathway to glucose production in the body.

Here is another clue that tells us the body does *not* want to remain in the ketogenic state long-term: Even *one* higher-protein meal can kick you out of ketosis. Why would that be the case? It seems the body prefers to waste precious protein to make glucose, even though it is an energetically expensive and somewhat toxic process (ammonia is released when amino acids are "de-aminated") that requires extra energy to deal with.

As you can see, ketosis is great for survival, but is not an *optimal* state to be in; certainly not in the long term. It requires an Olympic level of mental gymnastics to believe and argue otherwise.

"But the science, Christian, the science!"

Before you whack me over the head with the hundreds of studies that have shown the ketogenic diet to be "safe and effective™" for this or that, let me tell you that most of them were short term—in the region of one to three months. We can design any number of experiments that show short-term benefits from an intervention. The human body is so resilient that most anyone could plod through the couple of months of a keto trial. Heck, many of us have been running on stress hormones for much of our adult lives! In addition, studies were done with athletes, bodybuilders, and CrossFitters—those folks will take an exorbitant amount of punishment before they notice deleterious effects. Short-term trials are useless in identifying long-term negative effects of the ketogenic diet.

Furthermore, a massive confounding factor exists in many of the studies: the substantial weight loss in the participants. If you are overweight and lose, say 15kg (33 lbs), that is going to exert multiple positive effects on your health. Your blood pressure, lipids, and glucose will improve. Your joints, heart, and cardiovascular system will be less stressed. You (and possibly your partner) will sleep better and that alone could be life-changing. The list goes on. As I explained in the last chapter, the increased circulating fat in conditions like obesity, metabolic syndrome, and type-2 diabetes is a major causal factor in insulin resistance. Decrease the person's body fat stores and they will become more insulin sensitive, which will enhance their overall metabolic function.

So next time someone tells you that keto cured their Aunt Mary's diabetes, ask them how much weight she lost, because invariably that played the biggest role (along with improving the quality of the diet). While I will acknowledge that there are many anecdotal reports of people curing their cancer or auto-immune condition with a keto diet, it is hard to overstate what a big confounder weight loss is in the clinical trials. Also, in those miraculous recoveries, it is likely other factors played a role besides the keto diet, such as removing toxic processed food and improving lifestyle factors that were contributing to the illness.

Finally, and this really irks me, a lot of diet studies mainly look for improvements in "cardiometabolic" markers such as cholesterol, blood-glucose, HbA1c, and so on. Those get lowered, and everybody is high-fiving each other because we showed the keto diet "reduced cardiovascular disease risk". Yay. Please hand me the puking bucket. The truly valuable markers to monitor during these studies are the sex, adrenal, and thyroid hormones such as testosterone, DHEA, cortisol, adrenaline, TSH, T3, and so on. But they are rarely reported because (surprise, surprise) the keto diet tanks the protective hormones and raises the stress hormones.

Keto will decrease your metabolic rate over time

Going back to what I said earlier, if your body is receiving the signal that it is in starvation mode, which is what carbohydrate restriction does,[2][3] it will gradually start to shut down non-vital functions. You may meet the occasional person who has been doing keto a long time (though it is likely they get in-and-out of ketosis regularly), but they will invariably be relatively young, very healthy, and lead a pristine lifestyle with a high-quality diet. While I still do not think it is the *optimal* approach for their long-term health, it's hard to convince those folks of that when they feel and perform well. Perhaps if they checked their hormones more often, they would be more receptive.

However, if you start from a relatively poor state of health, it is likely you'll experience the negative effects on your metabolism sooner. For a stressed person who is loaded up with PUFAs and follows a sub-optimal diet and lifestyle, several months can be enough to cause serious damage.

It is striking how quickly your body starts slowing down its metabolism when you cut out carbohydrates or abstain from food (again, they both send a similar signal). But it makes complete sense, as you would not survive a famine for long if you kept up your regular metabolic rate several days into it! The body acts quickly because that is what will ensure its chances of survival. Researchers have shown that even *four days* on a ketogenic diet (without a reduction in calories) results in a significant fall in the active thyroid hormone T3:

> **The hormonal pattern switched towards a catabolic mode** with a fall in insulin levels (-44.0 +/- 6.3%) and a **rise in glucagon** concentration (+39.0 +/- 10.4%). A significant **fall in triiodothyronine** [T3, active thyroid hormone] and rise in reverse triiodothyronine were observed, while thyroxine levels remained unchanged.[2]

"Catabolic mode" means breaking down the body. Many of us have been led to believe that a reduction in thyroid hormones, testosterone, or other protective factor after experiencing a stressor is to be expected, and our bodies bounce back stronger due to the hormetic effect of fasting, exercise, and other "mild" stressors. That may be the case if you are young and healthy, but when we're chronically stressed, we gradually lose this ability to bounce back—thus adding more stress to our plate only makes things worse. The body is quick to lower the metabolism, but is slow to ramp it back up, which is why recovering from metabolic dysfunction can be a slow and frustrating process. Just ask anyone that has destroyed their metabolism from dieting or a long-term low-carb diet, and you will see your metabolic rate is something you need to protect at all costs.

A study on the ketogenic diet in children with epilepsy, published in 2017, is a disturbing example of the risks. After one month on the diet, eight children were diagnosed with hypothyroidism. At three months, seven more were diagnosed, and at the six-month stage, another five were determined to be hypothyroid. Twenty of the 120 children, or about 16%, were put on thyroid medication within six months of commencing a ketogenic diet.[4]

The question is, were those twenty children in the study anomalies, or were the rest going to become hypothyroid at some point? My guess is that it was only a matter of time for many of them. Keep in mind that children, even with epilepsy—or autism, as has been my clinical experience—are more resilient than middle-aged adults that have been exposed to decades of stress, toxins, and PUFAs. So if the keto diet can make children hypothyroid, you can bet it will do the same in adults even more easily.

"But the Inuit eat mostly seal blubber and they are fine!"

You will sometimes hear that the Inuit (Eskimo) traditionally ate a very low-carbohydrate diet, proving that humans can survive with little to no carbs for generations. Again, the keyword here is *survive*. Were they thriving, though? Would they have eschewed carbohydrates if they were readily available all-year-round? From what I have seen, the Inuit life expectancy is 10 to 15 years shorter than the average Canadian, which doesn't make them the most convincing example of the wonders of a low-carb diet.

The argument may then be, "That's because they are eating more processed sugar and other spoils of the modern world." Okay, but their life expectancy *has* been increasing steadily, just not as much as Canadians' has, and the gap is enormous.[5] If any of this ancestral stuff made sense and the thesis that "low-carb is healthier" is correct, then the Inuit should have started out as living longer and their life expectancy would decline after the introduction of the processed carbohydrates and other crap. But basically, the opposite happened. Or, if modern advancements that increase life expectancy permeated their society, they should now live longer than the average Canadian because they eat more fat and less carbohydrates than the rest of us.

I understand that living up in the North is tough; there are struggles these folks go through that could contribute to their shorter life expectancy. But that proves the point that they have to do various suboptimal things out of necessity in order to survive. Not eating carbohydrates was one of them, simply because they were unavailable. The takeaway here is: We should not assume that what people did to survive in the past is optimal (or even necessary) for our long-term health today—especially given how drastically different our modern environment is.

What is interesting about the Inuit is that they have a mutation in the CPT-1a gene, which impairs their ability to create ketones. This means they were not in ketosis even when eating only meat and seal blubber. The fact that this genetic variation survived to this day indicates that chronic ketosis was not the most favourable state for the survival of those living in the Arctic. My hunch is their shorter life expectancy may be in part due to their increased need for glucose production via gluconeogenesis, the stress of which causes wear and tear on the body that diminishes longevity.

Since we are on the ancestral thread, let's pretend the narrative that we evolved around the equator in Africa is indeed correct. That means fruit sugar was likely our primary source of fuel for millions of years. Sure, we may have migrated to Northern climates where the seasons prevented us from having year-round carbohydrate sources, but that was after a long time of subsisting on fruit and whatever we could hunt or scavenge.

The fact is that humans have genes for carbohydrate-digesting enzymes like maltase, sucrase, and amylase (a starch-digesting enzyme present in our saliva and made in the pancreas). This is clear evidence we were munching on fruits and starches throughout much of our history. Some low-carb proponents argue that the body makes all the glucose it needs through gluconeogenesis, and we do not need any exogenous carbohydrates sources. Why, then, do we produce various carbohydrate-digesting enzymes in the body?

When we zoom out on human history even a tiny bit, it is evident that we were already consuming large amounts of sugar and grains for centuries and millennia before the advent of the current chronic disease crisis. Can someone please explain to me how we managed to avoid obese children, adolescents with diabetes, young adults with autoimmune diseases, or people in their forties developing cancer or early onset Alzheimer's until the last century? Maybe climate change is a causal factor today... Yes, that has to be it.

Sugar seems to be a convenient scapegoat to take attention away from the true culprits: seed oils, ubiquitous use of herbicides and pesticides, thousands of other toxic chemicals in the environment, air pollution, and ever-increasing levels of radiation. Not to mention the unprecedented levels of psychological stress, lack of sunlight, exposure to too much blue light at night, and iatrogenic (induced by medical activity) causes of debilitation.

As I mentioned already, I avoid grains in my diet and advise my clients to do the same if their goal is optimal health and longevity. They are far from ideal foods to consume regularly. I also do not advocate for the use of processed sugar, especially in the context of ultra-processed junk food. But if we look at it objectively, civilisation as we know it was made possible by the mass cultivation of grains. Sugar practically fuelled the Industrial Revolution, which is only half-joking. Carbohydrates are **not** to blame for the chronic disease epidemic.

I have also heard certain keto proponents say that entering the ketogenic state once in a while is super-healthful because our ancestors did it. Why? Where is the evidence that our ancestors were healthier because of that, or that we can be healthier by doing it? It sounds like another one of those unverifiable evolutionary fairytales that we are just supposed to believe. There are (for now) still plenty of healthy people in their eighties and nineties that got there without fasting or going into ketosis periodically. We have evidence that it is possible to live to a hundred and beyond while still smoking or drinking and eating bread and sugar, but we don't have any evidence of low-carb or keto-centenarians.

"I'm just using the ketogenic diet to lose weight."

There is a common misconception that keto is a magical fat loss tool, as if eating a high-fat diet somehow defies the laws of thermodynamics. Aside from the impressive weight loss in the first couple of weeks—which is mostly water and glycogen—the primary reason folks shed pounds on a keto diet is because it helps them achieve a caloric deficit. That's it. A high-fat diet is more satiating than a high-carbohydrate diet and that allows you to eat less. Further, since a ketogenic diet doesn't allow bread, chips, and most processed garbage, you are forced to eat more *real* food. Who wouldn't feel substantially better doing this?

I can't blame those who have experienced such "newbie gains" for becoming fanatical about the diet and defending it as if it's their religion. But if we evaluate it objectively, the "magic" of keto weight loss comprises eating whole foods and consuming fewer calories than you expend. Not exactly rocket surgery. The fact is, if you maintain a caloric deficit, any diet will help you lose weight, at least initially—it does not matter if it is low-fat, high-protein, or even just pizza and doughnuts. Not that I'm saying it's simply about "calories in, calories out", because hormones play a major role in the weight loss equation (though few people understand this aspect, hence their weight-loss attempts are often ineffective).

As an example, a 2022 Cochrane review of 61 randomised-controlled trials (with almost 7,000 total participants) that compared low-carb and balanced carbohydrate diets' efficacy in reducing weight and "cardiovascular risk" concluded that:

> There is probably little to no difference in weight reduction and changes in cardiovascular risk factors up to two years' follow-up, when overweight and obese participants without and with T2DM [type-2 diabetes] are randomised to either low-carbohydrate or balanced-carbohydrate weight-reducing diets.[6]

When observed through a more-nuanced lens, low-carbohydrate diets appear to be nothing more than an allopathic tool—they are a symptom-reducing tactic rather than a long-term solution to the problems of excess weight and blood sugar dysregulation. The quick weight-loss and improved blood glucose *markers* give the impression that success has been achieved regardless of whether or not the person is truly getting healthier. We all love short-term solutions, but deep down, we know quick fixes suck. You may lose weight faster with keto, but because your metabolism will be lowered, regaining the pounds will be as easy as *thinking* about a slice of strawberry cheesecake. Then, when Thanksgiving and Christmas come along, you're screwed.

To be clear, I do not recommend dieting of any sort, but… If one were to decide to do it, it actually appears that restricting fat is superior to restricting carbohydrates for the purpose of fat loss. This was observed recently (but also in lots of prior research) in a study titled, "*Calorie for Calorie, Dietary Fat Restriction Results in More Body Fat Loss than Carbohydrate Restriction in People with Obesity.*"[7] The participants of that trial were confined to a metabolic ward, which is a unit specially designed for nutrition research where they can't leave during the duration of the experiment.

Locking people up in a ward helps prevent them from sneaking in candy bars or running to the convenience store to load up on snacks, so as not to skew the study results. Every meal they eat is prepared and meticulously quantified in terms of macronutrient content. They are watched over as they eat to make sure no one is cheating, and a researcher accompanies them to the bathroom to make sure they don't throw up anything and that their poops are kosher. Okay, that last part was a joke, but they *are* watched over when they have visitors to prevent anyone from smuggling in a balloon filled with M&Ms up their rectum. Prison conditions, essentially. But it's for Science™, so let's trust the process.

The study in question found that carbohydrate restriction led to an average of 53g of fat loss per day, whereas fat restriction resulted in an average of 89g per day of fat loss[7]—a massive difference. What this tells us is that the greater relative weight loss (compared to low-fat or balanced carb diets) experienced at the initial stages of low-carb diets is probably due to the increased stress they cause (less dietary glucose causes the body to break itself down at a faster rate). That paper was published in 2015, but it has been known for decades that a high-fat diet predisposes a person to weight gain much more so than a high-carbohydrate diet. Here is a quote from a paper published in 1995:

> Metabolic studies show that diets high in fat are more likely to result in body fat accumulation than are diets high in carbohydrate. There is no indication that simple sugars differ from complex sugars in this regard.[8]

Somehow, we've been conditioned to think that as soon as your lips touch something sweet, you're off to the races storing up fat and giving yourself diabesity type-8. In fact, it is much is easier to store fat than to convert glucose to fatty acids. When you eat some butter, enzymes in your gut break it down into the individual fatty acids that are then absorbed into the intestinal cells. There, they get repackaged back into triglycerides, then into chylomicrons, and finally are absorbed into the lymphatic system and sent down various pathways in the body. At that point, storing them is easy—all you need is a fat cell to pick them up. Turning glucose into a fatty acid involves more steps, and as the authors of the paper quoted above said:

> It would be intuitively surprising if humans routinely undertook the biochemically expensive process of fat synthesis from carbohydrate when they have an abundance of preformed fatty acids available from their diet.[8]

They also stated:

> There is ample reason to associate high-fat diets with obesity but, at present, no reason to associate high-sugar diets with obesity.[8]

If you are still not convinced that a low-fat diet is more conducive to weight-loss than a high-fat one—don't worry, it also took me a while to come around to the idea—let me ask you this: When researchers want to induce type-2 diabetes in lab animals, do they use a high-fat or a high-carbohydrate diet? I've had a fun time asking people this question lately and invariably everyone says that they would use a high-carb diet. Nope!

Fun fact: Researchers use a *high-fat* diet to make animals insulin resistant, and subsequently diabetic. It is an incredibly reliable method that takes but weeks to achieve the goal.[9] A 60% fat diet is enough to do the trick, though I am sure the high-PUFA content of those lab diets speeds up the process. But the point is: If sugar is so fattening and low-carb diets are so great for health and weight loss, why does the standard protocol to induce diabetes in rats use a high-fat diet? As Matt Damon said in that movie about the guy with the thing about a dog, "How about them apples?"

Is the ketogenic diet worth doing if you're healthy?

Some folks tell me they're on the keto diet for "health purposes" or to improve their performance. While mimicking starvation to enhance your performance is quite the oxymoron, it is true that studies with obese individuals have shown improvement in inflammatory markers. We must, however, keep in mind that those results are very likely to be confounded by the weight loss accompanying ketogenic diets. Conversely, one four-week study of healthy young men on a very low-carbohydrate diet showed no considerable changes in markers of inflammation, so it's doubtful a longer period would have shown much of any benefit.[10] If your health is in good nick, perhaps you're doing some things right. Why mess with a diet that is untested in the long-term and—did I mention this already?—is designed to *mimic starvation*?

Too often, people conflate the "benefits" of keto with simply removing inflammatory foods from their diet. Case in point: If you cut out hard-to-digest grains, beans, lentils and other fibrous plants, you're likely feel better. Your gut lining will get a break from the onslaught and as it heals, your immune system will dampen its activity. This will lower inflammation and reduce the growth of certain types of bacteria that thrive on indigestible-for-you fibre.

Beautiful things will then happen: You may sleep better, have more energy, a better mood, and your poops will smell of roses. Eating a high-fat diet wasn't the thing that did it, though—it was removing the lectins, starches, and fibres. If you had swapped out the crappy carbs for easy-to-digest cleaner alternatives like honey, fruit, maple syrup, and organic white rice, you could have experienced similar benefits without the risk of slowing down your metabolism. But doing that is not as sexy as posting on Instagram about how epically my keto diet is going, so it is kind of a non-starter.

Let me recapitulate the case against keto: The ketogenic diet mimics starvation and will lower your metabolism (which is bad for many reasons). The primary reason it is effective for weight loss is because of the caloric restriction afforded by the increased satiety of meals high in fat. The removal of processed and chemical-laden foods is a major reason many folks feel amazing on it. Studies showing benefits are often done with athletes or obese populations and are too short in duration to show the long-term deleterious effects of sending your body the signal of starvation. Weight loss is a massive confounding factor in trials with overweight individuals that showed benefit from the ketogenic diet intervention.

In summary: *Yeah, that's gonna be a no for me, dawg.* But anyway, since being in ketosis long term is difficult to maintain, you may opt for the easier "low-carb" approach. This strategy is just as misguided.

Why low-carbohydrate diets suck royally

I know, I know. Johnny down the street won an Ironman triathlon and finished his PhD while volunteering at the local animal shelter, all on a low-carb diet. It saved his marriage. His boss promoted him. The Pope sent him a Christmas card with a $50 gift voucher. Let's set aside anecdotal reports, impressive as they may be, and let's simply review the *mechanisms* at play in the body when carbohydrates are restricted but we do not enter the ketogenic state.

Soon after your last meal, your blood sugar will start to fall. Your stress hormone system will kick in to pick up the slack until the next time you eat. Except your next meal will not contain much or any carbs. You are already creeping into Stress Mode. Gluconeogenesis continues in the liver and uses protein from your meal to make glucose. Over the next few days, glycogen in your liver and muscles is gradually depleted. Stress Mode gets turned up.[11]

Any time your blood sugar drops, stress hormones are elevated even further to ensure you can continue functioning. While the liver is busy cranking out glucose, cortisol signals your muscles, bones, and organs to break down to supply substrate for gluconeogenesis. A lot of the protein you eat is "wasted" by getting converted into glucose instead of being used to repair and rebuild your body. That is, unless you eat a high-protein diet, but that adds a burden on your kidneys and has been shown to result in a drop in testosterone.[11]

If you decide to do some exercise (been there, felt the pain), you can bet cortisol will shred even more of your lean tissue to make sure you have enough glucose to sustain the activity—rather counter-productive, as you're robbing Peter to pay Paul, where Paul is the muscles the exercise targets, and poor Peter is the lean tissue in your body that was broken down. After all this self-cannibalisation, your post-exercise cortisol will remain elevated for longer than it would have otherwise, as research has found:

> Resting and post-exercise cortisol increase during the first 3 weeks of a low-carbohydrate diet. Afterwards, resting cortisol appears to return to baseline, whilst post-exercise cortisol remains elevated. High-protein diets cause a large decrease in resting total testosterone (□ 5.23 nmol/L).[11]

Does that sound *anything* like a state conducive to good health, much less optimal performance or longevity? If you said no, good for you. You get a gold star; now go have a snack and take a nap. It raises my cortisol just thinking about doing a fasted workout ever again.

While the research does not consistently show that low-carb diets result in lowered testosterone (age, health status, and study duration being big confounders), you can expect your androgen levels to decline, eventually. This is to be expected when cortisol is high because it opposes testosterone. Evidence for this is the fact that when people are injected with cortisol, their testosterone levels decline.[12]

> Testosterone (T) is the primary male sex hormone, and vital for reproductive development and function. Moreover, low endogenous T is associated with an increased risk of chronic disease, including type 2 diabetes (Yao et al., 2018) and cardiovascular disease (Corona et al., 2018). In many respects, cortisol is biochemically opposed to T, as the administration

of exogenous cortisol lowers T[11]

Decreased testosterone is deleterious in women, too. And I'm sure I don't need to remind you that all that extra cortisol is driving ageing and disease:

> Similarly, the reverse relationship between cortisol and chronic disease risk is observed, with higher levels being associated with an increased risk of cardiovascular disease mortality[11]

To sum up: low-carbohydrate diets increase cortisol and can reduce testosterone; both of which are associated with disease. At least when you get into ketosis, the brain can use ketones to function and that spares glucose for other organs and tissues while taking some burden off the liver. On a low-carb diet, however, it's only fatty acids and glucose that provide the substrate for energy production. And since the brain doesn't burn fatty acids, you're in quite the metabolic pickle. Your poor liver will need to work overtime.

Most people need at least 200-250g of carbohydrates per day

You would think I wouldn't need to put in such effort to convince people of the importance of carbohydrates for optimal performance and longevity. Low-carb proponents go as far as to call carbohydrate a "non-essential" nutrient because the body can synthesise glucose on its own. While technically true, there are plenty of compounds that are considered non-essential because our bodies can produce them, but that does not mean excluding them from the diet is conducive to optimal health.

It seems more plausible that we have multiple ways of making glucose in the body *because* it is so freaking essential! After all, we have a complex system of hormones that will do almost anything to make sure our blood sugar remains in range. We will literally break down our bones, joints, organs, and muscles to give the liver substrate for gluconeogenesis. That's how important glucose is. It's so critical to survival that the first thing you get put on if you have a serious accident and land in the emergency room is a glucose drip—otherwise, you'd fall into a coma and soon die.

Let's do some rough back-of-a-napkin calculations. Researchers estimate that the brain consumes about 120g of glucose per day.[13] When we factor in the red blood cells, which need around 30g of glucose per day, we're already at 150g. As you can see in Table 6, a 50kg (110 lbs) woman consuming 40% carbohydrate in her diet would barely cover just these basic requirements. Of course, you're not vegetating on the couch all day, so you'll need more glucose than that—how much depends on your weight, activity levels, and metabolic rate.

Now imagine you are on a diet that provides only 75g to 100g of carbs. How do you think your body will deal with the glucose deficit? If you said stress hormones and gluconeogenesis, you are correct. And if you decide to go for a brisk walk or a weights session at the gym, what gets cranked up? That's right, cortisol. Of course, by the end of the session, the adrenaline and endorphins will have given you a pleasant buzz, so you will feel great and think you "hit the spot" with that workout. Keep doing that week in, week out for a decade or two and you are bound to get in trouble.

I hope you now understand that all but the tiniest of us need at least a couple of hundred grams of carbs per day just for basic functioning, and that number increases dramatically if you're active. Use Table 6 as a rough guide to see your ballpark figures.

Table 6: Carbohydrate requirements based on Mifflin-St. Jeor equation and light activity level (15-30 minutes of elevated heart rate activity, one-to-three times per week)		
Characteristics	**40% carbohydrate**	**55% carbohydrate**
Female, 50kg (110	164 grams	226 grams

lbs), 50-yrs, 165cm, 25% body fat		
Female, 65kg (143 lbs), 50-yrs, 165cm, 25% body fat	186 grams	256 grams
Male, 80kg (176 lbs), 50-yrs, 180cm, 20% body fat	246 grams	339 grams
Male, 100kg (220 lbs), 50-yrs, 180cm, 20% body fat	276 grams	379 grams

How to increase your carbohydrate intake

Alright, let's say I've convinced you that low-carb is not the way to go, or you now realise that even though you were not "low-carbing", increasing your intake is prudent. You've put away your over-sized "LOOK AT ME! I'M ON A KETO DIET!" badge and have cancelled your weekly baker's dozen order of Kerrygold butter. What's next?

If you've been on a low-carbohydrate diet for months or (heaven-forbid) years, you probably don't want to suddenly start eating 300g of carbs a day. As you may have developed some level of insulin resistance, it is best to increase your intake gradually while reducing fat proportionally (assuming you were eating a sufficient amount of calories).

As I alluded earlier, the cleanest carbohydrates are honey, maple syrup, fruit and fruit juice, because they don't contain the anti-nutrients that plague cereals, grains, beans, and legumes. Milk is also a great source of carbs, protein, and plenty of other nutrients if you tolerate it well. Organic white rice—the one exception as it comes to grains—is one of the best choices to use with savoury main meals, but you can also indulge in the occasional sweet or white potatoes. Not that other carbs are completely off the table—as long as you do not rely on them as daily staples and you're not afflicted with gut or autoimmune issues, occasionally partaking in guilty pleasures is fine. Like I said, if we keep the crap out of our homes, we've done the most important part.

While you can do it any way that works for you, my favourite carb additions are 30-60 minutes before bed and first thing in the morning. Before you say, "I can't do that, it's incompatible with my intermittent fasting regime," I'll say that your intermittent fasting regime is not compatible with your health and longevity goals!

Longevity tip: Break your morning fast soon after you wake up

By the time you wake up, you've been running on your backup system for hours. Because you weren't moving, it's easily manageable for your body. But as soon as you get up and start going about your day, your glucose requirements increase considerably. The *last* thing you want to do is continue running on the backup system because you will soon be in Stress Mode. What's the point? To burn some extra fat? That whole notion is bunk. You will be burning mostly lean tissue, mediated by increased cortisol levels, *and* ageing yourself faster.

Since a lot of us, myself included, don't want to eat a full breakfast first thing, you can break your fast with some organic honey, maple syrup, organic fruit or juice. When I say *some*, I don't mean a few sips or a teaspoon of honey, okay? I am talking about a full glass of juice, or two to four tablespoons of honey. We're not messing around here. Your poor liver is close to depleted of its glycogen stores, of which it can hold around 100g. If a glass of juice is about 30g of carbs and three tablespoons of honey contain 50g, you will be far from topped up. The idea is to add fuel, so the breakdown of your body is halted. Doing this is doubly important if you like to start your day off with a cup of coffee. Because caffeine is a central nervous system stimulant, it will rev up your metabolism. If there is no fuel to burn for energy, guess what gets used?

Since your tank (liver) is nowhere near full yet, you need to have a balanced meal soon—ideally within an hour. By balanced, I mean just that—each macronutrient needs to be represented. The reason to include all macronutrients in all main meals is straightforward: carbohydrates spare protein (so you don't need to convert it to glucose and burn it for energy), fat spares carbohydrates (for the brain and nervous system, as muscles burn fat at rest) while increasing satiation and keeping you full for longer, and the protein is essential for building and repairing everything in the body (and it also helps with satiation). All are essential and excluding any of them for prolonged periods signals a stress state to the body that we want to avoid.

Please note that if you feel an energy slump after the honey top-up, it does not mean that "carbs are bad" and I am talking nonsense. It probably means your stress hormones—which were propping you up—were lowered, thus you experienced your current "baseline" state. It's akin to stopping coffee cold-turkey—the first few days can feel pretty horrible if it was the crutch keeping your energy levels up. If this does happen to you, understand you have been running in Stress Mode for a while and this adjustment, as uncomfortable as it may be, is for the betterment of your long-term health.

Longevity tip: Top-up your liver glycogen stores before bed

They say, "never go to bed angry", I say: Never go to bed hangry. My go to is to use three-to-four tablespoons of organic honey to give my liver fuel, about an hour before bed. It works well for many of my clients too, because it is a quick and tasty solution with minimal preparation or cleanup. Honey or maple syrup is a jumping off point, of course. You can use whatever clean carbohydrate source you prefer. If your dinner was within two hours of your bed time and you ate sufficient carbohydrates, you may opt for less honey. You will learn what works best for your body as you experiment with it. For example, if I wake up in the middle of the night and it takes more than a few minutes to fall back asleep, the first things I consider are: did I eat enough carbs near bedtime and should have I had more, and is the room temperature too warm or too cold?

Doing the honey top-up is particularly important if you eat dinner 3-4 hours before your bedtime. In this instance, especially if it was a fairly low-carb meal, your liver is going to kick into glucose-production mode within an hour or two of you falling asleep. This means your stress hormones will soon rise and that may cause you to wake up and have trouble falling back asleep. I've had clients whose sleep issues were completely and permanently resolved just by trying this simple hack.

"Is honey before bed going to make me fat and diabetic?"

Excuse me while I scream into a pillow... Ah, much better. I hope by now you understand that going to sleep does not mean your physiology suddenly shuts down. Your brain, liver and other organs continue working and consuming glucose. If you're staying reasonably active throughout the day, your muscles' glycogen stores will also need replenishing after the liver has had its fill.

But here is the part that most of us find counterintuitive: when cells have "surplus" energy, they do not just store it. Think about it this way: let's say you get a promotion at work, and they raise your salary by 20%. Are you just going to stuff that extra cash in your mattress and forget about it? Virtually no human in the history of the world has done that. You may decide to replace the fridge with a newer model, or to renovate the kitchen, or otherwise invest the extra income in something that will make your life more comfortable or entertaining.

It is the same when the body has more energy. When a cell receives extra fuel and produces more energy, it can use it to repair DNA, rebuild its membranes, and fuel countless other regenerative processes. (I could swear that once I transitioned to a higher carbohydrate diet, my eyesight improved.) Sure, if we eat more than our body needs, we will store the excess as fat, but as I discussed previously, it is way easier to store fat than to turn glucose into fatty acids. Even if you consume 300-400g of carbohydrates per day—an ungodly amount to those who have been sold the low-carb ideology—*de novo lipogenesis* (the creation of fat from glucose) will be *negligible,* as long as you eat close to your caloric requirements.

> Indirect calorimetric measurements indicate that exceptionally high intakes of carbohydrate are required before the respiratory quotient exceeds 1.0 (a value indicative of net fat synthesis)[8]

For a somewhat exaggerated example of how little excess dietary carbohydrate is stored as fat, let's turn to an overfeeding study where the subjects ate 50% more than their caloric requirements as either only fat or only carbohydrate for two weeks. During this undoubtedly unpleasant for the participants experience, the researchers measured how much of the excess energy was stored. This is what they reported:

> **Carbohydrate overfeeding** produced progressive increases in carbohydrate oxidation and total energy expenditure **resulting in 75-85% of excess energy being stored**. Alternatively, **fat overfeeding** had minimal effects on fat oxidation and total energy expenditure, leading to **storage of 90-95% of excess energy**. **Excess dietary fat leads to greater fat accumulation than does excess dietary carbohydrate**, and the difference was greatest early in the overfeeding period.[14]

Even with obscene amounts of carbs—I can't even imagine having to eat an extra seven cups of cooked rice (1500 kcal or about 375g of carbs) per day for two weeks straight—up to a quarter of the excess was not stored. What do you think happened to that 15-25% of energy? As expected, the participants' metabolic rate increased:

> With carbohydrate overfeeding there was a significant increase in energy expenditure on days 7 and 14[14]

If you overeat fat, 90-95% of it will be stored on your body with almost no increase in your rate of fat-burning or overall metabolism. Conversely, as you add more carbs to your diet, your metabolism keeps increasing (to a point), which carries the regenerative benefits I touched on above.

> It is generally accepted that dietary carbohydrate promotes its own oxidation, whereas dietary fat does not (16-19). This was clearly the case in the present study. Fourteen days of fat overfeeding produced no significant changes in fat oxidation or total daily energy expenditure.[14]

What's interesting is that the researchers thought that the energy storage caused by the carbohydrate overfeeding was mostly because of inhibited fat oxidation (i.e., there was so much glucose coming in that it inhibited the use of fatty acids for fuel), and not from turning carbs into fat! Here is what they said:

> Although the issue of whether carbohydrate overfeeding led to de novo lipogenesis in tissues such as the liver cannot be definitively determined in this study, **the calorimetry data indicate that net lipogenesis from carbohydrate did not occur.** There were short periods during some carbohydrate overfeeding days in which the nonprotein RQ was > 1 .0, suggesting that some de novo lipogenesis occurred. It is impossible under conditions of this study to accurately quantify this de novo lipogenesis. **Other investigators using isotopic techniques have reported that de novo lipogenesis in human subjects is not a major way to accumulate body fat stores** (28). It may, however, be slightly higher in hypeninsulinemic obese subjects than in lean subjects and may depend on the type of carbohydrate in the diet (29). **From these results, however, we conclude that positive fat balance was due to a decrease in fat oxidation accompanying the increase in carbohydrate oxidation.**[14]

My point here is that you have nothing to worry about adding an extra 100-200g of clean carbohydrates to your diet. As long as you balance it with a proportional decrease in fat (roughly reduce 50g of fat for every 100g of added carbs, if eating close to caloric requirements), provide the B-vitamins and other co-factors needed to turn the carbs into energy (which meat, liver, and egg yolks will provide), and are reasonably metabolically healthy, you should expect to see improvements in energy, mood, sleep, and libido, much of which will translate into in-creased longevity.

Conclusion

Neurons are largely intolerant of inadequate energy supply, and thus the high energy demand of the brain predisposes it to a variety of diseases if energy supplies are disrupted. A large variety of central nervous system pathologies are the consequence, and sometimes also the cause of disturbed cen-tral or peripheral glucose energy metabolism, which can be affected at almost every level of the cellular or biochemical metabolic cascades[15]

Remember this and tell all your low-carb friends: we don't just create fat out of carbohydrate willy nilly. It's an energetically expensive process that the body avoids, especially when pre-formed fatty acids are coming in from the diet. Yes, eating too much fat and carbs together is conducive to putting on weight, but the weight gain will come mostly from the dietary fat being stored. And while carbs will increase insulin and that is a stor-age signal, if we keep dietary fat moderate and don't overeat, it should not be a problem.

Since we won't find any long-lived people who subsisted on low-carb or ketogenic diets, we'd have to wait decades for data to accumulate on whether eating this way affects longevity posi-tively. My hunch—based on anecdotal reports of hypothyroid-ism and infertility of those who went low carb—is that the risk of long-term metabolic dysfunction outweighs any short-term benefits.

5. Signal Abundance to Your Body — Part 2

Contrary to popular dogma, as usual, fasting of any kind and calorie restriction are *not* conducive to longevity because they send the highly stressful signal of scarcity to your body.

Let's define a few terms before we explore these topics. Fasting, also known as water fasting, is the practice foregoing food for 24 hours or more. Intermittent fasting (IF), also called time-restricted eating (TRE) or feeding (TRF), is the practice of limiting your daily food consumption to a window of time. A common format is eating during an eight-hour period and fasting the other 16 hours (16/8). If you are extra-primal, you could go for the 20/4 format, or even the OMAD version where you eat "one meal a day". (The MAD part of the acronym is quite apt because you'd have to be *loco* to think it's good for you.) Below is the thesis I will present to you.

- Fasting, intermittent or otherwise, is unnecessary if you eat high-quality *real* food and are metabolically healthy.
- If you have health issues and/or are under a lot of stress, fasting is going to be further stress that you do not need to add to your already burdened system.
- If your diet is terrible, full of inflammatory seed oils and processed foods, taking time off to fast may provide benefits, but there are healthier and less torturous ways to achieve them (like eating better food, for a start).

- If your gut is in rough shape, there are ways to address the issue without starving your body of the fuel and nutrients it needs to heal itself.
- Intermittent and water fasting lowers your metabolic rate, which makes it easier to gain weight in the long term if you continue eating the same amount of calories. Neither are ideal weight loss strategies.
- Caloric restriction, or dieting, is deleterious because it also lowers your metabolic rate, increases cortisol, and forces your body to cannibalise itself to survive.

With all the rage that intermittent and water fasting have become in recent years, you would think there is solid science backing their purported benefits. But alas, even a cursory search for studies of the wondrous power of starving yourself for most of the day (or, God-forbid, multiple days) reveals little but dubious animal experiments and scant human research that actually shows plenty of detrimental effects from these interventions.

I will readily admit once again that I was on the bandwagon. Intermittent fasting was doable, but I could not manage more than two straight days without food. Even a 36-hour fast felt lousy; I would spend most of the time on the couch feeling sorry for myself. Perhaps fasting while on a low-carb diet was extra bone-headed of me... You live and learn! Armed with hindsight and a slightly more nuanced understanding, I now see little value in starving myself for any length of time. And given the precarious state of health of much of the population, I would not recommend that most anyone engage in it.

First, let's examine the evolutionary argument for fasting: our ancestors did it, so it must be good for us! This old chestnut again. The question we should ask is, why did they fast? Logic would make me think it was almost always because there was a lack of food, not because they wanted to "upregulate cellular autophagy" or some special anti-aging pathway a scientist discovered in a worm.

Moreover, we're told our distant ancestors lived much

shorter lives. How is their regular fasting an argument *for* longevity? If anything, it should be an argument *against* it! As for our more recent ancestors, historical records show they did not live longer than us either. Since injury and infection would have been among the most common causes of death back then, our advancements in technology (sanitation) and medicine (lowered infant mortality, antibiotics, and bordering-on-miraculous emergency care) play a big role in our increased lifespans.

However, let's not forget that we also have houses, supermarkets, and refrigerators in our age—and they are stocked full of food! (Or products purported to be food, in many cases, but that's besides the point.) Think about it: we're overfed and simultaneously under-nourished, and the sickest we've been in history, and with the highest pollution levels, and unprecedented levels of stress, and poisoned by agri-chemicals and medical drugs. Yet, our life expectancy is still higher than our ancestors'. Something does not add up with the "fasting for longevity" narrative.

I've learned that, just like the ketogenic diet, it's imperative that we evaluate statements like "our ancestors did X, so we should also do it" through a more critical lens, lest we be suckered into lighting our barbeque by bashing rocks together. Our predecessors chewed on raw tubers dug out of the ground to extract some barely palatable carbohydrates. They endured bee stings to enjoy the delicious honey they plundered and feasted on rotting carcasses. They often put their lives at risk hunting or gathering hard-to-reach foods. (Apparently, falling from trees was a leading cause of the death back then.) Emulating things they did out of necessity—not because they were optimal for their health—is clearly madness. Do you think if your cave-dwelling great grand folks had a fridge full of fresh fruit and meat, they would fast out of their own volition for even *one* day out of the year? I doubt it. Chronic disease like we see today did not exist back then, so it's unlikely they were using water fasts to cure their diabetes or autoimmune conditions.

We also have to factor in the things our ancestors had going well for them: all their food was organic and wild-caught, there was no pollution or plastics, they walked barefoot and slept on the Earth, were naked in the sun all day, and had orders of magnitude less stress than we do today. Maybe fasting for a few days in those conditions would have been fine. You could chill in the sun while waiting for others in the tribe to return from a foraging or hunting expedition. You wouldn't have had to worry about your job, inflation, World War 3, an alien invasion, or Elon Musk putting a chip in your brain. Today, overzealous folks go on a multi-day fast without even taking time off work, and they think they're doing their body good…

But Christian, what about all the research showing fasting and calorie restriction as being the best ways to increase life- and healthspan? Are you a science-denier?!

Why research on fasting and caloric restriction is (mostly) bunk

Ah yes, the research. Forgive me for being brash, but a lot of it is pure garbage. You and I could have come up with better studies after a night out of doing tequila shots. You would be appalled at how much poorly designed, low-quality research gets pumped out every year. Your tax dollars fund a significant portion of it, too. Now, I fully agree that the people conducting the experiments are highly intelligent and well-meaning. But too often, their hands are tied because their research sponsors call the shots. If those folks want an outcome that will support their agenda, they'll find ways to get to it. We should not be so naïve to think it won't happen in science, especially when we know that companies selling symptom-masking chemicals for profit are often involved. Please understand that I'm not criticising the fine folks that ran the studies, but the system within which it all takes place. It is dogmatic, agenda-driven, and financial gain is often the sole motive.

So it is with longevity research. Certain factions are adamant that calorie restriction and fasting are the golden ticket to increasing lifespan, so they'll push that narrative and focus mostly on the positive findings in their studies. They will rationalise away or simply ignore negative findings. Mainstream media will pick up the studies and roll with it. Once public opinion is shaped, it can take decades to undo the conditioning; meanwhile, untold damage will be done to the populace. (A prime example is the decades-old cholesterol and heart disease theory that just won't die because billions of dollars in annual revenue are at stake.)

In any case, let me present some facts and you can be the judge on whether we should blindly Trust the Science™ on fasting and calorie restriction for longevity.

Most research into lifespan extension starts with so-called "model organisms". These include worms and fruit flies and allow for theories to be tested inexpensively before investing resources in experiments on higher animals. The tiny nematode *Caenorhabditis elegans* (*C. elegans*), measuring about 1mm, is a commonly used organism to test hypotheses such as caloric restriction as it relates to increasing lifespan. And studies show that it works. Hooray! Let's all start skipping lunch post haste.

However, what we're not told is that when *C. elegans* senses that there is insufficient food in its environment (or other stressors), it enters a suspended state (called *dauer*) which is akin to hibernation. It can survive in this state for multiple months, whereas its normal lifespan is only about a month. So that completely invalidates *all* of that work in terms of its transferability to humans.

But don't you worry, we have tons of other animal studies showing caloric restriction and intermittent and prolonged fasting improve health and increase lifespan. A few have even been done with monkeys! And since in the eyes of the Science™, you are basically a glorified monkey, this research clearly shows you need to eat less food and you will live longer.

There is just one small bone I want to pick with the research… That is the "food" the animals eat during the experiments. To say their diets are a disgusting concoction of toxic slop would be an understatement. The standard lab rat chow is a mix of soybean meal, fish meal, corn and soy oil, synthetic vitamins, and "might-as-well-have-ground-up-some-rocks" for minerals. It's similar for monkeys and other mammals.

Now, do you think if an animal eats less of this processed garbage, or is forced to fast intermittently or for prolonged periods, it might have better outcomes than its counterparts eating their regular diet? I think so, especially because often the control groups in the studies are allowed to eat as much as they want, known as *ad libitum* feeding. Those animals tend to overeat and become fat, which predisposes them to metabolic complications and further health problems. Then, when a study compares the fat and sick control group to the calorie restricted or fasted experimental group, the latter is shown to be healthier and live longer. Well, no shit, Sherlock. While not every study has this massive confounding factor, many do—which invalidates them as evidence that restricting food intake extends lifespan.

I don't know what these unfortunate animals did in their past lives to deserve the torture they're subjected to. Bred in captivity, living imprisoned, fed toxic slop, blasted with fluorescent lights, handled, prodded with needles, and finally killed and dissected. But maybe they were research scientists in their previous lives, so they kind of deserve it? In all seriousness, the conditions lab animals live in are more suited to studying how the effects of stress and horrible diet cause diseases normally only found in humans. Case in point: In one of the major studies on caloric restriction in rhesus monkeys, one of the poor creatures died of what they diagnosed as systemic lupus erythematosus.[1]

> The second DR monkey, which died at age 23 years, was diagnosed with systemic lupus erythematosus (SLE). In humans, this chronic inflammatory disease of connective tissue is classified as an autoimmune disorder that affects the skin, joints, kidneys, nervous system, and mucous membranes. In

> this primate, the clinical situation presented as inappetance, anemia, leukopenia, decreased activity, generalized muscular atrophy evident in the limbs, and decreased range of motion, particularly in the rear limbs.[1]

Would you please tell me what the heck a monkey is doing developing lupus? Do you think monkeys in the wild are going to the monkey doctor and getting diagnosed with monkey lupus or macaque cardiomyopathy or simian "colonic adenocarcinoma (a cancerous tumour) with metastases to the liver and mesentery"? Because that is what monkeys in this study were dying of.

I admit I'm not an expert on this and I understand these animals have to die of *something* eventually, but I'd be much more inclined to think factors in their environment were contributing to these diseases. Perhaps it was climate change. Perchance it was some weird Science™ stuff they were doing to them (one monkey died the day after receiving ketamine for an experiment (what?) and two others' deaths were anaesthesia-related). Or maybe, just *maybe*, it was their diet.

You would think for a study this long and important, they would feed the control group a set amount of calories to control for the confounding variable of *ad libitum* (AL) food intake. Nope.

> The AL-fed monkeys were provided the diet in an amount that allowed for food to be readily available 24 hours/day and which allowed each monkey to determine its daily intake on an individual basis.[1]

This trial took decades to complete and probably cost a bazillion dollars—how could they allow such a fundamental flaw to taint the data? They handicapped the control group from the outset, so it's no wonder the calorie-restricted group did better overall. As you can see, there is a lot more nuance to these studies than the sexy sounding soundbite "caloric restriction and fasting increase lifespan". Here is a final quote from the paper:

> The oldest primate in the current study (Monkey L-9; a female rhesus), which **was also maintained on ad libitum feeding**, lived to the remarkable age of **40 years old**. She had been diagnosed with type 2 diabetes mellitus at age 29 years and, therefore, was maintained on insulin therapy for approximately 11 years.[1]

How ironic is that? The oldest living monkey wasn't even part of the caloric restriction group! Great sciencing, guys! The paper stated that although she was diabetic and had limited vision, "she was otherwise in excellent health, physically active, and alert even at her advanced age". Isn't it shameful how in our age you can be in "excellent health" despite having limited vision and having to take insulin for your diabetes?

It's interesting that while insulin is often vilified—allegedly causing diabetes and obesity and everything in between—it is what kept this monkey alive for an extra 11 years. My theory on why it helped this tortured soul live so long is because insulin opposes stress hormones like glucagon and cortisol—when it increases, they decrease. Less cortisol means less destruction in the body, hence slower ageing and degeneration. Does that mean we should all go to our doctor and demand an insulin prescription? Why would you, when you could just eat your clean carbs?

If we *truly* want to understand whether fasting or caloric restriction extends life- or healthspan, we need to feed lab animals an organic diet that more-closely resembles their one in the wild—eggs, insects, nuts, meat, and so on. Supplemented nutrients should be in the high-quality forms found in products sold for human consumption. No mineral oxides or carbonates. And of course, no seed oils. Then, we need to keep the animals' external stresses to a minimum and at least attempt to replicate some of the positive conditions in nature, such as correct circadian timing (e.g., rats are nocturnal), exposure to sunshine, and reduction of fluorescent light and radiation.

Then, after we have baseline data on how long the animals live in these slightly more optimal conditions, let's start limiting their food intake and putting them on various fasting protocols. My hunch is the animals will do better on a standard diet that approximates their caloric requirements (not *ad libitum*) because it will keep cortisol and other stress hormones lower than all the fasting and food restriction protocols. Not that this type of research will ever get funded…

Longevity tip: Reduce your intermittent fasting window

An overnight fast of ten-to-twelve hours is plenty for most people (especially for those over the age of forty). Anything past that and you are bound to be running in Stress Mode. Don't be a hero. The few grams of extra burned fat are not worth it. Even a rudimentary understanding of the physiology of starvation—which is literally what fasting is—should dissuade most people from engaging in this madness.

What happens when you fast

The mainstream fairytale: When you fast, magical pink unicorns descend from the heavens and shower you with autophagy and hormesis. You are delivered from your sins. Your karmic debt is repaid, as decades are added to your life…

Now for the real-world version.

Since a similar physiological response is initiated during fasting as when reducing your carbohydrate intake (that is why the ketogenic diet mimics starvation), we'll only briefly review the first part. A few hours after your last meal, your liver takes over the job of maintaining your blood sugar by secreting glucose from its stores. As its glycogen stores decrease, stress hormone secretion increases, which stimulates gluconeogenesis and the breakdown of lean tissue and fat stores.

Your activity level determines the intensity of these processes. If you rest on the couch (the smartest move), your heart and muscles will burn fatty acids for energy, sparing the created glucose for the central nervous system (which includes the brain). If you get up and start moving, your glucose demands increase significantly, causing gluconeogenesis to rev up. By now, you understand that this is facilitated by stress hormones. Because your body is now in survival mode, it halts many repair and regeneration processes and the building of new proteins.

Wait, don't I go into ketosis and all is well? Not exactly; ketosis happens much later. You certainly won't be in ketosis when intermittent fasting, and should you decide to suffer through a three-day fast, it's likely half of that time you will be running primarily on gluconeogenesis as you deplete your body's glycogen stores.

Here is a rough estimation of how much of the day you would be in Stress Mode on a 16/8 IF regime. Let's say dinner was at 8 p.m. and your next meal will be at noon the next day. Depending on how much food you ate at dinner (and especially how much carbohydrate), your glucagon will rev up by around midnight to signal your liver to begin breaking down its glycogen. As those stores get depleted, cortisol and other stress hormones gradually increase.

Once you wake up, say at 6 a.m., and start moving, your stress hormones elevate even more to mobilise substrate for energy production. Should you decide to indulge in a cup of coffee or two in the meantime, a further rise in stress hormones will ensue. By noon, you could easily have been running in Stress Mode for the past six hours (and potentially for longer, if dinner was light or your glycogen stores were depleted for other reasons). During this time, if you feel shaky, lightheaded, hangry, or irritable, understand it's caused by hypoglycaemia and the hormonal responses to it. The same is true if you feel great, "high", or elated. Throwing in a fasted workout or cardio session before lunch will place an even greater burden on your body to maintain your blood glucose level during the activity.

There you have the basic gist of it. Perhaps you burned a

little more fat than you would have otherwise, but you also sacrificed a substantial amount of lean tissue, facilitated by cortisol. Hence, you also aged yourself. If you think I'm only "theorising" here, let's see what some of the research that is not widely publicised has found.

Intermittent fasting lowers your metabolic rate

A study showed that it takes as little as **two weeks** (!!!) of intermittent fasting to lower resting energy expenditure (REE) significantly in lean, healthy people. A lower REE means a lower metabolic rate. That is bad, in case it wasn't clear by now. It means your body is burning fewer calories than before, which means some functions got turned down or off. The study authors concluded:

> The decrease in resting energy expenditure after IF indicates the **possibility of an increase in weight during IF when caloric intake is not adjusted.**[2]

Right, so I have to reduce my calorie intake on the intermittent fasting regime, otherwise I risk gaining weight in the longer term. That makes sense. Sign me up. Did I mention this decrease took only *two weeks*? The researchers estimated the median decrease in REE at about 59 kcal per day. Over the course of a year, that equals 21,535 kcal, or about 3 kg of body fat. Let me make sure I understand this: I go on an IF regime, it quickly drops my metabolic rate, and now I have to decrease my food intake in order to not gain weight. If I don't, I will gain in the order of 3kg of body fat in a year. Perfect. But at least I'll live longer—right, guys? Guys?

Time-restricted feeding is ineffective for fat loss and causes loss of lean mass

"But intermittent fasting is helping me lose weight!" you might say. Is it, though? Or is it the reduced caloric intake due to the difficulty of stuffing down three full meals and a snack in an eight-hour period? As one 2020 paper in *JAMA Internal Medicine* stated:

> Time-restricted eating, in the absence of other interventions, is not more effective in weight loss than eating throughout the day.[3]

That is kind of disappointing. But the devil in the details, which wasn't clearly mentioned in the paper's abstract (the only part most people read), was that the **TRE group lost lean mass in their trunk and limbs**, while the normal diet group did not. The researchers (or perhaps their editors) wrote:

> There was also a significant difference in appendicular lean mass index between groups (-0.16 kg/m2; 95% CI, -0.27 to -0.05; P $=$ .005).[3]

Pretty vague. I guess it was bad news enough that TRE without deprivation is useless for weight loss. Adding insult to injury by clearly stating you may lose precious lean tissue would have been too damning of this intervention that has become one of the darlings of the health and fitness world. Digging into the paper, the authors said:

> In analysis of secondary outcomes, **we found a significant reduction in lean mass in the TRE group.** In the in-person cohort, **the average weight loss in the TRE group was 1.70 kg. Of this, 1.10 kg (approximately 65% of weight lost) was lean mass; only 0.51 kg of weight loss was fat mass**. Loss of lean mass during weight loss typically accounts for 20% to 30% of total weight loss.[3]

Before you say, *"Some loss of lean mass is always expected when losing weight,"* compare the study outcomes with what the average lean mass loss is normally:

The proportion of lean mass loss in this study (approximately 65%) **far exceeds** the normal range of 20% to 30%. In addition, there was a highly significant between-group difference in ALM. Appendicular lean mass [lean mass in the limbs] is correlated with nutritional and physical status, and **reduced ALM [appendicular lean mass] can lead to weakness, disability, and impaired quality of life**. This serves as a caution for patient populations at risk for sarcopenia because **TRE could exacerbate muscle loss**."[3]

One last quote from the paper:

Finally, the extent of lean mass loss during weight loss has been positively correlated with weight regain.[3]

There you have it. Intermittent fasting can lead to muscle loss in your limbs, which can lead to weakness, disability, and reduced quality of life. And, because losing muscle (which is metabolically active tissue) lowers your metabolic rate, you are at risk of regaining the weight. Funny how there was no mention of this study on the Wikipedia page about intermittent fasting when I last accessed it. Apparently, the doctor that conducted this trial immediately stopped his intermittent fasting regime after seeing the data, and told his patients to do the same. In a CNBC article, he said, "Just losing weight alone doesn't mean good things are happening for your health."[4]

You know what I found amusing? When I retrieved the article in November 2023, there was a link to a video at the bottom of the page that was titled, wait for it: "How this CEO lost 80 pounds with intermittent fasting." The comedy writes itself.

I hope now you see why I advise my clients to reduce their fasting window, especially women and those older than forty. Muscle is difficult enough to gain and maintain—you don't want to give your body *more* reasons to let go of it. Another factor that can decrease your muscle mass is a drop in your testosterone level, which brings us to the next point.

Intermittent fasting lowers testosterone in men and women

A review of human trials on the effects of IF on reproductive hormone levels in females and males showed that testosterone was lowered in both. The authors said:

> As for men, **intermittent fasting reduced testosterone levels in lean, physically active, young males**, but it did not affect SHBG concentrations. Interestingly, muscle mass and muscular strength were not negatively affected by these reductions in testosterone.[5]

The biggest risk I see with interventions that lower your protective hormones without an immediate physical manifestation of such, is that it can lull you into a false sense of security. Then, months down the line, when your libido is in the tank and you are struggling to muster up the motivation to get out of bed, you may suspect the culprit to be parasites, mould toxicity, toxic metals, EMFs, or perhaps evil spirits. This can cause people to chase their tail looking for the problem when it was simply prolonged Stress Mode causing all manner of havoc in their body.

But don't fret, it's not all bad news. A paper titled "Twelve Months of Time-restricted Eating and Resistance Training Improves Inflammatory Markers and Cardiometabolic Risk Factors" must bring good tidings, right? Sure, if you just read the abstract.

> Our results suggest that long-term TRE combined with a resistance training program is feasible, safe, and effective in reducing inflammatory markers and risk factors related to cardiovascular and metabolic diseases[7]

Safe and effective™, hey? Heard that one before… While they did not lie, this is another nauseating example of chasing "cardiometabolic" markers, as if lowering cholesterol actually lowers the risk of heart disease. But what's particularly frustrating to see is the authors glossing over the reductions in testosterone. The TRE group in this study saw a staggering drop—almost 17%—in their total testosterone by the end of the 12 months. The most striking thing when you look at the data was that much of this decline occurred after two months. A similar eight-week TRE study was published by the same research group where there was a comparable drop in testosterone.[7] This tells us that lowered testosterone appears to be a feature of TRE, rather than an occasional anomaly.

In summary, intermittent fasting lowers your metabolic rate, will lower your testosterone, is not effective for weight loss on its own, and will cause you to lose precious lean tissue. However, please remember that it is not so much the studies that we need to rely on, but the basic understanding of the physiological mechanisms at play that allow us to "survive" periods without food. To reiterate, these mechanisms are facilitated by our stress hormones, which are destructive when chronically elevated. Understand that and you will be well equipped to discern what is beneficial and what is detrimental for your health. Intermittent fasting clearly falls in the latter category.

Longevity tip: Skip the water fasts entirely

In a world of logic and common sense, if intermittent fasting lowers your metabolic rate and testosterone and up-regulates your stress hormones, surely it goes without saying that water fasting will do the same—times a bazillion. And yes, research has demonstrated that fasting results in an elevation of the stress hormones such as adrenaline, (epinephrine), noradrenaline (norepinephrine), cortisol, growth hormone, glucagon, and serotonin, and a decrease in insulin and thyroid hormones (T3 and T4).[8-10] So far, so bad.

Now, let's see what a gruelling multi-day fast will do to you. In our first example, one study found that a 10-day fast (with 200-250 kcal per day in supplemental nutrition) in men resulted in an average weight loss of close to 6kg, with about 40% of it being fat mass. What about the other 60% of lost weight? Around 58% of that was water and glycogen stored in the liver and muscles, while the other 42% was what the authors termed "metabolic active lean tissue"—also known as 2.5kg of liver, kidney, heart, intestine, and muscle tissue, broken down primarily to produce glucose![11]

The fast also reduced the participants' basal metabolic rate (BMR) by 12%, which is to be expected because muscle is highly metabolically active, and the body lowers the metabolic rate as a survival mechanism during starvation.

Keep in mind the study subjects were allowed 20g of honey, a glass of organic orange juice and another of vegetable broth daily that provided about 200-250 kcal of nutrition. That certainly spared tissue their bodies would have sacrificed to keep them alive. Without this supplement, the loss of lean mass could have been significantly greater than 25%, because 250 kcal is roughly 62.5g of glucose—easily an extra 100g of lean tissue lost each day. That approximates another 1kg (2.2 lbs) of lean mass loss over the duration of the study. Yikes. All other factors being equal, it would have meant a one-to-one loss of fat and lean mass; not exactly the results I'd want from a "health" intervention.

What seemed particularly sadistic in this experiment was the added "1 h gymnastic group class including whole-body stretching and yoga, and outdoor walks for 30 min in the morning and 90 min in the afternoon". Talk about adding injury to injury. The last thing you would want to do when starving is exercise. It does, however, demonstrate how much punishment the human body can endure (and how misguided we can be in terms of what we think are healthful practices).

The study participants may have been pleased to see their waist circumference reduce by 4-5cm during the fast, but it had returned to baseline in the follow-up three months later. As far as strategies to fit into your wedding suit go, I think we can relegate this one to Plan B. To their credit, I'm glad that the authors stated the following near the end of the paper:

However, given the popularity of fasting seen in public media, we obviously urge extreme caution when applying fasting in **underweight** or **older individuals**, as well as in patients with eating disorders, patients who are **suffering from higher severity or end-stage chronic diseases** and those **taking medication** that may be impacted by fasting, or patients undergoing chemotherapy who are more vulnerable to sarcopenia.[11]

In other words, don't fast (at least that is what I understand by "extreme caution") if you are underweight, are older, have an eating disorder, or have cancer or a higher severity chronic or end-stage disease. That list doesn't leave that many people that are eligible to fast. It seems like you need to be in the Goldilocks zone of being eighteen-to-sixty years of age, not underweight, without severe chronic or end-stage disease, and should not be on medication that may be affected by fasting.

The question is, should you fast if you are obese or have type-2 diabetes? While we probably can't classify these conditions as "higher severity" in most cases, I would posit that most people in these states aren't exactly a picture of health. They are likely to have a lot of stored PUFAs and toxins in their adipose tissue, as well as multiple nutrient inadequacies or deficiencies that will be worsened by fasting. Their stress levels are likely to be high and their livers may be dysfunctional, given how common non-alcoholic fatty liver disease (NAFLD) is nowadays. My view is that those folks shouldn't fast either, because the reduction in metabolic rate and loss of lean mass will probably cause more harm in the longer term than the short-term benefits provided by the fast.

Put simply, you *can* fast if you are relatively young and disease-free. But if you are young and healthy, what the hell is the point of fasting? Well, there is something that it can help with…

Fasting will shrink your balls

Are your testicles, or those of your partner, the size of tennis balls? Gross! Are you sick of everyone constantly staring, and not being able to find pants that fit comfortably? Well, worry no more, you freak, because we have just the intervention you need to shrink those pesky *huevos* back down to a more manageable size...fasting!

A paper titled "Eight Days of Water-Only Fasting Promotes Favorable Changes in the Functioning of the Urogenital System of Middle-Aged Healthy Men" (or, as I believe it should have been titled, *"How to castrate men without actually castrating them"*) reported that after eight days of water-only fasting, the men's total testicular volume decreased significantly (about 17%), along with decreases in total and free testosterone, and dehydroepiandrosterone (DHEA), while sex-hormone binding globulin increased significantly. And, get this, they had the gall to conclude that:

> These results indicate that 8 days of water-only fasting improved lower urinary tract functions **without negative health effects**.[12]

Are you having a laugh? Who was running this study, Dr. Mengele from the Depopulation Department? Shrinking testicles and reductions in the protective hormones testosterone and DHEA are EXTREMELY negative health effects—it just takes time for them to manifest as outward symptoms. And that is what a lot of these studies fail to account for—the long-term consequences of the interventions. The researchers pat themselves on the back for reducing X or Y marker (often completely irrelevant ones too) and move onto the next experiment.

I'll tell you, when I was at my worst in terms of libido and low energy (due to the parasites), my testosterone was in the region of 619 ng/dL, and I felt absolutely horrible. The mean testosterone level of the participants prior to the fast was just under 600 ng/dL (594.89 ng/dL $\pm$ 216.58). After the eight days it was 385 ng/dL ($\pm$ 167.65). That is a 35% decrease. Free testosterone decreased by 27% and DHEA by 22%. The conclusion of this study should have been "Fasting decimates men's gonads and should never ever, not ever, be engaged in, for any purpose, whatsoever." Or something to that effect. What's mind-boggling is how throughout the paper, the authors were lauding the amazing benefits of the procedure:

> Taking into account the positive changes in the results of the uroflowmetry test, the volume of the testes and prostate, metabolic and reproductive hormones related to the urogenital system, and the improvement of the quality of life of the studied men after 8 days of water-only fasting, **systematic use of caloric restriction or the use of intermittent or continuous fasting of short duration should be considered, as a method of prophylaxis or health therapy.**[12]

Right. Thank you. I'll file fasting under F, for "Freaking Never". Seriously, remind me again why starving ourselves is beneficial. Ah, yes, of course. The Holy Grail. The kiss from Zeus. The Philosopher's Stone. Autophagy.

What about autophagy?

If you've somehow missed the news of the wonders of autophagy and how it's the best thing since sliced cheese, let me catch you up. The term comes from the Greek *autophagos*, which means to "self-eat". It is the process that we are told is upregulated when we fast and is supposedly beneficial because our cells are forced to recycle parts of themselves that are not in optimal condition. The marketing slogans are along the lines of "cellular rejuvenation" that is the key to your vibrance, performance, healthy ageing, and longevity. All very scientific. "It" won the Nobel prize, after all, don't you forget that! (That is how I've seen it promoted, honestly.) Well, so did the guy that came up with the lobotomy procedure, so let's not get too excited...[13]

An enquiring mind should ask: *Why* does fasting upregulate autophagy? What is triggering this process to be increased inside our cells?

If you look up another term, *apoptosis*, which is a kind of "cell suicide" (programmed cell death), you will see that one trigger for a cell to commit apoptosis is **glucose deprivation**. When cells sense a lack of glucose, knowing they will soon become dysfunctional, they dismantle themselves in a coordinated fashion so the body can use their parts for the greater good (much of which will be to produce glucose for the starving organism). Apoptosis is a tidier way for a cell to die, as unintentional death can lead to inflammatory processes that are detrimental to the organism. Another trigger for apoptosis is the binding of cortisol to the glucocorticoid receptors. In plain language, a lack of glucose and other stresses cause cells to commit suicide. Not to say that autophagy and apoptosis are the same thing, but this is what specialists in these areas are saying:

> Autophagy is active in all cells and can be upregulated in response to stress or nutrient deprivation.[14]

And:

> ...it is generally accepted that autophagy functions as a mechanism to survive cellular stresses like nutrient deprivation...[14]

So it appears that both autophagy and apoptosis are upregulated or triggered by stresses such as nutrient deprivation. In other words, starving yourself will increase autophagy because cells are nutrient or glucose deprived. Do you see where I'm going with this? Maybe my sweet marketing slogan for autophagy will make it clearer: "Starve yourself to upregulate the process that is caused by starving yourself!" Pretty catchy, huh?

Don't get me wrong, both of these are vital processes that are running all the time to a degree. I just don't think we need to go out of our way to increase them, especially because starvation upregulates "non-selective" autophagy, which, as the name suggests, targets not just redundant proteins and damaged or aged organelles (which is what "selective" autophagy targets), but also healthy parts of the cell. Again, this is because when you don't eat for a prolonged period, it's a major state of emergency in the body (even though you may not perceive it as such), hence it prioritises making glucose to stay alive at the expense of a lot of cells being dismantled and lean tissue getting broken down.

> Autophagy is a process that targets various intracellular elements for degradation. Autophagy can be non-selective — associated with the indiscriminate engulfment of cytosolic components — occurring in response to nutrient starvation and is commonly referred to as bulk autophagy. By contrast, selective autophagy degrades specific targets, such as damaged organelles (mitophagy, lysophagy, ER-phagy, ribophagy), aggregated proteins (aggrephagy) or invading bacteria (xenophagy), thereby being importantly involved in cellular quality control.[15]

And look, even if I am completely off-base and increasing autophagy is so super awesome, remember that a lot of other bad stuff is happening while you fast. Cells (which are part of tissues that are part of organs) are dying left and right because of glucose deprivation. Others are being voluntarily broken down to turn their components into glucose. It is in no way an optimal state of being, and the fairytales that "the body rebuilds better and stronger" afterwards are just that—tall tales with little to no substantiation. Let's see follow-up data from human study participants and how their health markers look in one, five, ten years and beyond, and then we can talk again. And not just their "cardiometabolic risk profiles", but their thyroid, sex, and adrenal hormones and various inflammatory markers—i.e., actually useful data.

The bottom line is that forcing autophagy by putting your body in Stress Mode does not seem like it's essential for longevity—in fact, it looks to be counterproductive. And if you *really* want to upregulate yourself some autophagy (it sounded right in my head), just go do some exercise, because that has also been shown to do the trick.[16] But again, no need to overdo it, because it is a stress and survival pathway, after all.

The benefits of fasting

Surely there are *some* benefits to fasting. There are countless reports of people healing various diseases and we can't discount these anecdotes. But again, let's not conflate losing weight during an intervention as the benefit *of the* intervention. If weight loss was what contributed the most to the healing, there are healthier ways to accomplish the result without sacrificing 25-30% of the lost weight as precious lean tissue and facing the dire consequence of a lowered metabolic rate. Not to mention the potential organ and vascular damage caused by increased circulation of PUFAs and toxins stored in the fatty tissue.

If the benefit of fasting was the break the person had from their processed and highly inflammatory diet, that means we can replicate the benefits largely by removing the junk and replacing it with real, organic, whole foods.

And if the benefits of fasting were due to the lowered inflammation and dampened immune response caused by a gastrointestinal imbalance, we have ways to address gut issues (some of which I'll discuss later) without starving our bodies of the much-needed nutrients and energy they require to heal.

Longevity tip: Don't diet!

Don't restrict calories. Don't skip meals. Don't give your body a reason to turn down its metabolic rate. Eat real food—

organically grown or raised, pastured or wild-caught. It's exceedingly difficult to overeat chronically when you eat wholesome meals you have cooked yourself. Calorie restriction is unlikely to extend your life, and if you feel you need to lose weight, there are healthier strategies to do it. If dieting worked, at least half of overweight people would be slim because they have tried it. Instead, they can't sustain the deprivation and when they stop, they often gain extra weight because the restrictive period wrecked their metabolism. This is no way to live.

I already addressed the problems with calorie restriction research in animal models—namely the terrible diet the poor creatures are fed and the fact that they are often compared to *ad libitum* control groups that overeat and get fat, causing them health problems. The ridiculous part is how little actual effect caloric restriction (CR) has on increasing lifespan when started later in the life of lab animals:

> The benefits of CR, however, decline as the age of onset of treatment is delayed. Modeling these impacts suggests that if a 48-y-old man engaged in 30% CR until his normal life expectancy of 78, he might increase his life expectancy by 2.8 y.[17]

Assuming we could even extrapolate the animal research to humans, if a 48-year-old man cuts his caloric intake from 2500 to 1750 kcal per day and were to sustain this level of restriction for the next 30 years, he might expect a life extension of about 2.8 years. Gee, where do I sign, Satan?

Worse even, if the same person started the calorie restriction regime seven years later, at 55 years, the extension is modelled to be only an extra six weeks. Six weeks! But don't worry, I used my sophisticated modelling algorithm to estimate that those six weeks will actually feel like six years due to the suffering imposed by being hangry all the time. Science™ to the rescue! *You're welcome, starving man. Enjoy your increased longevity.*

It's important to note that researchers have shown the life-extending effect of caloric restriction may be because of the reduction in PUFA consumption—though we have little hope this information will make it to the mainstream. Cell and mitochondrial membranes that have less PUFAs are more resistant to oxidative damage, which slows down the ageing process.

For example, one mouse study had three groups that were on 40% CR diet with the fat sources coming predominantly from soy, fish oil, or lard (pig fat).[18] The control group was on a 5% CR soy diet and as expected, those animals had the shortest lifespans. What's interesting is that the CR fish oil group had the least life extension, while the CR soy group was in the middle. The lard group's lifespan saw the longest extension. However, as may you recall from chapter two, because pigs are fed so much corn and soy, their fat is quite high in PUFAs. Most conventional lard can easily contain as much as 20% PUFAs, and in this study, they stated it contained 15% linoleic acid (the predominant omega-6 fatty acid). So this was in no way a low-PUFA diet! If they had used butter or coconut oil, I can almost guarantee those mice would have lived even longer.

Nevertheless, studies like this show how beneficial PUFA reduction is for increasing lifespan. The longest-lived lard mouse in this study lived 112 days longer than the longest-lived mouse in the other groups—a vast increase for these animals. The researchers concluded:

> The results of the present study indicate that dietary fatty acids influence life span in CR mice. In particular, a diet with a high proportion of monounsaturated and saturated fatty acids promotes a longer life span in CR animals maintained at a common energy intake (8.6 kcal/d) than diets containing a high proportion of unsaturated fatty acids.[18]

With that said, the reasons to not diet go deeper than it being an ineffective strategy for life extension. Not only will cutting calories lower your metabolic rate and thyroid function (which will make regaining the weight extremely easy), it will increase your cortisol and all its destructive effects on bone, muscle, and other valuable lean tissue. Not to mention feeling like crap all the time.[19] But that doesn't stop endless funding flooding this area of research. The following quote from a paper shows you how divorced from reality scientists can be:

> Therefore, bone loss at clinically important sites of osteoporotic fractures represents a potential limitation of prolonged CR [caloric restriction] for extending life span. Further long-term studies are needed to determine if CR-induced bone loss in healthy adults contributes to fracture risk and if bone loss can be prevented with exercise.[19]

Great, we know calorie restriction increases bone loss and risk of osteoporosis, so let's add exercise to the mix and raise stress hormones even more. That *might* prevent bone loss. How many PhDs did it take to come up with that stroke of genius? I guess they missed all the literature about stress and its effects on ageing and disease or cortisol's effects on bone. That is a big problem when you are focused in your tiny area of specialisation—you lose sight of what it means to be healthy in the real world. Everything boils down to mechanisms, statistical significance, and end-points. Little regard is paid to "insignificant" things like how a person would look, feel, and function on a 30% calorie deficit. How would they sleep? How will they interact with others? What will their quality of life be? None of these silly unquantifiable details seem to matter.

Bone loss occurs at a greater rate during dieting because the body is cannibalising itself to stay alive. A person stores 1kg or more of calcium in their bones. That will go a long way to keep vital functions going; but just because we *can* do this does not mean we should. You need to give your body the nutrients it needs daily, otherwise it either robs them of its less-important-for-immediate-survival parts or it begins to shut down non-vital functions, or both. This happens slowly, of course, so we can always chalk up any dysfunction or degeneration to "getting old" or genetics or bad luck. It could never be the fact that we're malnourished.

In keeping with the "most anything that makes it to the mainstream turns out to be useless or harmful" theme, calorie restriction not only won't help you live longer, it might actually send you to the grave sooner. If you dig around in the literature, you will soon find that **weight loss is associated with increased mortality** (i.e., incidence of death). Less surprisingly, weight fluctuation is also associated with higher mortality.[20-24] So, while we assume that excess weight gain is the big problem—it certainly does cause health problems and affects longevity—simply "losing a bunch of weight" only creates another set of metabolic complications that will shorten our lifespan. Here is another curious finding from the research:

> Evidence suggests that the highest mortality rates occur in adults who either have lost weight or have gained excessive weight. **The lowest mortality rates are generally associated with modest weight gains.**[25]

Why would losing weight or fluctuations in weight be associated with an increased chance of death, and why would a moderate increase in weight be associated with lower mortality? For one, it's because most people have not been taught how to lose excess weight safely. They do not realise how much stress and damage occurs during rapid weight loss that is mediated by reducing food intake, fasting, lots of exercise, and other popular modalities.

As discussed earlier in the book, we all have varying degrees of persistent organic pollutants (POPs) and other toxic chemicals stored in our fatty tissues. When we lose weight by cutting calories, we increase lipolysis, which sends fatty acids into our bloodstream along with whatever toxins those fat cells were sequestering. *No bueno.*

Intentional weight loss can increase health risk in the long-term, despite short-term benefits, because human adipose tissue is widely contaminated with various lipophilic environmental contaminants, especially persistent organic pollutants (POPs).[26]

If we add the release of PUFAs from our stores during weight loss to the POPs, we have a recipe for disaster as it comes to our thyroid function and metabolic rate (not to mention the inflammatory burden and other damage):

Clinical studies reported that POPs released during weight loss could negatively affect the resting metabolic rate, the oxidative potential of skeletal muscle, and thyroid hormone levels[26]

For an example of the short-term adverse health effects dieting can cause, let's turn to a study that compared a low-carb diet approach to a low-fat one. The estimated daily caloric intake was 1461.0 kcal (± 325.7 kcal) in the low-carbohydrate diet group and 1502.0 kcal (± 162.1 kcal) in the low-fat diet group, based on the participants' weight. Quite the restriction.[27] (How those poor folks sustained that for 6 months is beyond me—I'd probably land in the emergency room with an overdose of pizza and ice-cream by the second week, at the latest.) The low-carbohydrate group consumed around 29.5g (± 11.1g) of carbs, or 8% of daily energy intake, whereas the low-fat group consumed 197.6g (± 34.2g) of carbohydrates (52% of daily energy intake).

The study was sponsored by a low-carb advocate company, so as expected, the main conclusion was that the low-carb group experienced more weight loss (perhaps that is why only that group received a nutritional supplement during the trial). There was also, as per usual, some gobbledygook about the low-carb diet being "associated with a greater improvement in some risk factors for coronary heart disease"—you know the drill by now. What I found odd was how much more prevalent the reported adverse effects were in the low-carb vs low-fat groups:

- Constipation (68% vs. 35%)
- Headache (60% vs. 40%)
- Bad breath (38% vs. 8%)
- Muscle cramps (35% vs. 7%)
- Diarrhoea (23% vs. 7%),
- General weakness (25% vs. 8%)
- Rash (13% vs. 0%)

The question is: Why would people experience more rashes, headaches, general weakness, diarrhoea, and bad breath while on the low-carbohydrate diet? My immediate thought when I saw the data was that these are typical symptoms of toxicity or of the so-called "detox reaction" that occurs when a person releases more toxins than their body can comfortably handle (this often happens at the outset of a health-building program). This is precisely what I think these participants were experiencing.

Given their greater weight loss (i.e., much higher stress) than the low-fat group, they experienced increased lipolysis that caused more toxic compounds (and PUFAs) to be released into their circulation—hence the higher prevalence of adverse events. We can only speculate how much invisible and potentially long-term damage they did to themselves during this study. The low-fat group, having around 200g of carbohydrates per day, at least had enough fuel to run their brain and central nervous system. Of course, these were dismissed as "minor" events, but the authors also reported a more serious adverse event:

> One 53-year-old man in the low-carbohydrate diet group who had a family history of early heart disease developed chest pain near the end of the study, and coronary heart disease was subsequently diagnosed. During the study, this par-

ticipant lost 16 kg, his serum LDL cholesterol level decreased by 0.75 mmol/L (29 mg/dL), and his serum HDL cholesterol level increased by 0.21 mmol/L (8 mg/dL).[27]

I thought losing weight and decreased LDL cholesterol levels were supposed to make people healthier... They made sure to let us know about his family history of heart disease, though, so I'm sure this was all genetic and had nothing to do with the person having starved himself for months on end with stress hormones through the roof.

The truth is that *healthy* weight loss is one area where, unfortunately, there are no quick fixes. If you feel you are overweight and need to shift fat, you need to play the long game. It did not take a month or two to gain the weight, so you can't expect it to come off *safely* in a few weeks or months. Trust me. The price you will pay for dropping the pounds quickly will not be worth the (likely) temporary weight loss and worsened health status.

Focus on getting healthier and protecting your metabolic rate by following the advice in this book: Cut out PUFAs, eat real organic food, take your vitamin E, niacinamide, and other supplements we'll discuss, and add more walking into your day and keep gradually increasing it. You may also reduce your overall fat intake (e.g., to 15-20%) to stimulate your body to use more of its stores. If you can add regular sauna sessions to your routine to get the POPs out faster, that would also help. Work on building muscle (without over-stressing yourself) because it raises your metabolic rate and burns more fat when you are at rest. Then be patient.

While you're at it, look up the "obesity paradox" and you will see that being overweight or obese has been associated in some studies with a lower mortality rate in cardiovascular disease, cancer, and diabetes.[28-30] What that tells us, despite all the rationalisations in the medical community, is that storing excess fat is a protective mechanism for many people. In the case of someone with a serious hormonal imbalance or increased toxic exposure (including PUFAs) from their diet or environment, it is an infinitely better solution to store fat than to develop cancer, heart disease, or dementia.

My point is, we should not see excess weight as an enemy to defeat and banish. We must improve our health by fixing our metabolic issues and reducing all forms of stress that we can and focus on optimising our diet and lifestyle. When we do those things, our weight and body composition naturally start approaching the ideal numbers. "Losing a bunch of weight" is simply treating the symptom of metabolic dysfunction and often of a poor diet. Fixing food quality, stress factors, lifestyle, and metabolic blockages is addressing the root causes of the problem. As evidenced by the current disease statistics, reducing or masking symptoms is not the correct approach to resolve any chronic health concern, and excess fat gain is no different.

If you need personalised help with losing weight in a safe, sustainable, and stress-free manner, don't hesitate to get in touch with me through my website so we can accelerate the process together.

Conclusion

Your body works tirelessly around the clock—why starve it of the fuel and nutrients it needs to run the countless processes required to keep you alive and thriving? Why send it signals of famine? No reason, other than social programming, that we need to let go of. Eat high-quality food and provide your cells with plenty of their preferred fuel source (clean carbohydrates) and the nutrients they need to do their jobs. This is the most critical (though probably least sexy) component of a well-designed longevity plan because it will work wonders in keeping stress, inflammation, and oxidative stress (and the damage they cause) under control.

6. Nip Stress in the Bud

We've already done a lot to reduce your stress levels. Fuelling your body with sufficient clean carbohydrates, not skipping meals or fasting, reducing PUFA consumption, and improving your antioxidant status with vitamin E, all go a long way to protect you.

Fun fact: carbohydrates are so effective at reducing the negative effects of stress, that a study in the journal *Military Medicine*, titled "Effect of Carbohydrate Administration on Recovery from Stress-Induced Deficits in Cognitive Function: A Double-Blind, Placebo-Controlled Study of Soldiers Exposed to Survival School Stress" reported that:

> These data suggest nutritional interventions enhance the rapid recovery of complex cognitive functions impaired by exposure to significant or sustained stressful conditions. In addition to enhancing speed of recovery of function between operational intervals, the current data suggest that dietary supplement strategies may hold promise for enhancing field performance and a capacity to assist in sustaining operations by military personnel over time.[1]

The "sophisticated" nutritional interventions in the study were 6% and 12% carbohydrate beverages. If carbs are good enough to help recruits recover from "mock captivity" and "sustained psychological and physical stress during Survival School Training", you can be sure they'll help you keep stress hormones low. Don't be afraid to use this underrated but highly effective tool as a first line of defence.

Since ridiculous levels of psychological stress are inescapable in the modern world, we need to take it a step further. I'm going to give you a simple blueprint for reducing stress at the "nervous system level", so to speak. While using mindfulness techniques, meditation, breathwork, and the incredibly useful Emotional Freedom Technique (EFT) to counter stress and achieve a state of mental calm are viable options, I will present quick and easy solutions that require little work on your end.

But please remember that even though I can help you ameliorate some of the negative effects of stress, it's up to you to remove or reduce the sources of it that are within your control. You need to do this swiftly and aggressively because no amount of hacks or supplements will compensate for the damage caused by a stressful lifestyle. And please, don't go adding extra burden on yourself if you find the tools here work well for you. That's a classic mistake of the hard-charging go-getter, and a trap I've often fallen into. The golden rule should be: always try to reduce stressors, rather than add new ones to our life.

In my experimentation with dozens of supplements and techniques, I've understood what works for me consistently, but because we're all different, you may need to tweak the protocol to suit your body weight, stress levels, and other parameters. Always use the guidelines I give as jumping-off points and be ready to make changes based on how you feel. The goal is to avoid creating dependence on any compound and to avoid using sedation to "dull" the stress like a drug would. Rather, it's about helping your body "nudge" itself into the calm state or keep itself in it for longer. The way to do this is to use molecules that the body recognises. The beauty of this approach is that when you are in that state, external stimuli may be perceived as less stressful than they would be otherwise, and this allows you to respond in more productive ways.

We'll start with improving sleep because there is no better way to start the day than a restful, restorative night's shut-eye. You'll also need less coffee to get through the day. By the way, I find the whole notion of "getting through the day" repugnant. We should be "snapping necks and cashing checks" through the day, so to speak, not barely making it to "Netflix on the couch" time!

Sleep improvement tip: Use GABA to enhance your sleep

The amino acid GABA (gamma-aminobutyric acid) is the major *inhibitory* neurotransmitter in the body and is involved in reducing the excitability of neurons. It opposes the major *excitatory* neurotransmitter glutamate, too much of which can lead to excitotoxicity that can end in the death of brain cells. The inhibitory nervous system state is what we're looking to tap into to reduce stress.

Fun fact: you'll often find that when a herb, supplement, or drug has a calming effect, it is because it interacts with our GABA receptors in some way. These include benzodiazepine drugs, alcohol (though it has other effects in the body), and many plants. For example, the following herbs—known to have calming or sleep-promoting properties—contain various substances that modulate or activate the $GABA_A$ receptor:[2]

- Valerian (*valeriana officinalis*)
- Ashwagandha, Indian ginseng (*withania somnifera*)
- Chamomile (*matricaria sp.*)
- Passionflower (*passiflora incarnata*)
- Lemon balm (*melissa officinalis*)
- Schisandra, magnolia berry (*schisandra chinensis*)
- Moringa (*moringa oleifera*)
- Kava-kava (*piper methysticum*)

Isn't Mother Nature amazing? Here is the thing though: you

can buy GABA online, it's dirt-cheap, and it allows you to "cut out the middleman" because herbs, alcohol, and especially drugs may have undesirable effects. Herbs may contain impurities, contaminants, or compounds that have antagonistic effects to what you are trying to achieve. Alcohol can sedate, but it also dehydrates you, depletes nutrients, puts a burden on your detoxification system, and is too damn often frowned upon when used during the daytime and on the job. And drugs like benzos have "very occasional and totally mild" side-effects such as cognitive impairment, agitation, aggression, panic, negative withdrawal effects, and an increased risk of suicide. Hashtag Safe and Effective™. That's why I prefer to use amino acids and molecules that are not foreign to the body (with occasional exceptions).

How to take: Experiment with 100-1000mg of GABA 15-60 minutes before bedtime. The amount that works for you will vary, and more is not necessarily better. Even 300mg daily for four weeks improved not just subjective sleep quality in people with insomnia, but also objectively measured sleep efficacy (using polysomnography).[3] Not bad, given you can buy a six-month supply of GABA online for less than the cost of a mediocre bottle of wine. You want to start with a lower dose because too much GABA at one time can cause a slightly unpleasant (but harmless) tingling called paresthesia. If this happens, either lower the amount taken or take it with food, or both. You'll zero-in on the timing, amount, and whether with or without food works best for you in a week or two.

My current fail-proof sleep enhancement protocol is 300mg of magnesium glycinate with dinner, followed by 1000mg of GABA about thirty minutes before bed. This, along with my evening honey and making sure the room temperature is right, is usually enough to ensure I sleep well. It doesn't have to get much more complicated, but we'll certainly cover sleep improvement from different angles in future volumes.

GABA's usefulness does not stop with sleep. You can take it any time you feel the tension rising (or anticipate it to rise).

The trick with using it during the day is simply to use less because the bedtime serving *may* (but won't necessarily) make you sleepy (great if you want to take an afternoon nap, though). The brand I use comes in 500mg capsules, so if I decide to take it during the day, I use one capsule instead of the two I use at night. However, I rarely put myself into situations that elevate stress to a level where I feel GABA is called for, which goes back to what I said earlier: the more stressors you eliminate, the less supplemental "stress support" you'll need. In any case, the next supplement works perfectly during the day.

Stress-busting tip: Use L-Theanine in the daytime for its calming effects

L-Theanine, or just theanine for short, is an amino acid with a similar structure to glutamate (the excitatory neurotransmitter I mentioned above) that is found in the leaves of the tea plant (*Camellia sinensis*), and is the compound believed to give green tea the cognitive boosting properties without the jitteriness associated with caffeine. One possible mechanism through which it does this is by competing with glutamate for binding to glutamate receptors, thus inhibiting its excitotoxic effects and providing neuroprotection.[4]

Research has shown that theanine can reduce stress and anxiety, and improve cognitive function, mood and emotional status, sleep quality, and even blood pressure (which makes sense, given that stress raises our blood pressure).[5][6] Theanine is the ideal supplement for daytime use because it has a calming effect without causing drowsiness. It complements coffee superbly, helping you stay focused and productive without getting the shakes. (Don't forget to never drink coffee without sufficient carbohydrates in your system because it will increase stress hormone output.)

Theanine comes in 100-200mg capsules, but you can also

get it in powder form. Capsules are more convenient; just try to find a brand that doesn't use too many excipients. The brand I use contains only rice flour as an additional ingredient, with no silicon dioxide or other additives. If you plan to pair theanine with coffee, consider purchasing it in pure powder form as it's more cost-effective. Supplementing 200-400mg per day is an appropriate starting range to experiment with. I take it first thing in the morning on an empty stomach, followed by a further 200mg with every cup of coffee I drink (of which there were plenty during the writing of this book). Now that we have the basics covered, let's turn to one of my favourite supplements.

Longevity tip: Use pregnenolone for its calming, anti-inflammatory, and neuroprotective effects

The body makes pregnenolone from cholesterol—you know, the thing that's going to clog our arteries, kill us all, and possibly start World War 5. Yet somehow, by the grace of the good Lord, once we convert the abominable cholesterol to pregnenolone, it suddenly becomes beneficial in the body in a multitude of ways. Jokes aside, pregnenolone is actually the granddaddy of your steroid hormones such as testosterone, progesterone, estrogen, and even cortisol. It's also a precursor to various other protective *neurosteroids* that have some researchers all hot and bothered, and for good reason, too.

For a long time, pregnenolone was thought to be merely an inactive hormone precursor, which may be why relatively little research has been done with it. (Another reason could be that it's not possible to patent naturally occurring molecules, hence drug companies were not too interested.) This has allowed it to remain under the regulatory radar in some jurisdictions such as the USA, where it's available over-the-counter. Many countries allow its importation, though some don't—so make sure you understand the legalities of your region if you decide to implement it into your longevity program. And while I will share the products I use in the online appendix, always consult your practitioner before changing your diet or supplement program. While it is befuddling why slightly modified cholesterol (a compound our bodies produce) should require special permission to acquire in certain countries, it goes to show you how little concern governments have for their citizens' health and how influenced they are by the companies selling symptom-masking chemicals for profit.

Allopregnanolone: the miraculous metabolite

Here is where it gets even more interesting. When you take pregnenolone, it can be converted to *progesterone*, which plays various protective roles in the body to begin with. Progesterone can then be converted to *allopregnanolone*, which is an inhibitory neurosteroid that exerts its effects in part by potently acting on our $GABA_A$ receptors.

Allopregnanolone, or ALLO for short, has calming, stress-reducing, and sleep-promoting effects. You could even say it has anti-depressant effects, literally. So much so that the United States FDA (Food and Drug Administration) approved it in 2019 as a treatment for post-partum depression (PDD). And not just any PDD, but the "unresponsive to treatment" type, which is obviously really severe. And guess how many treatments are necessary to see meaningful results? Ten? Twenty? Nope, just one treatment is sufficient.[7] Of course, this is not a charity operation we're talking about, so that treatment is an expensive intravenous infusion with a disguised name (brexanolone) because why would you tell the people they can get the precursor (pregnenolone) to ALLO over-the-counter for the price of a Happy Meal?

How much does said treatment cost, you ask? Oh, only $7,450 per vial, which amounts to approximately $34,000 before discounts or insurance.[8] Does that include the cost of staying multiple days at the medical facility where the treatment is administered? *Of course not, freeloader. Where do you think you are, in a hippy commune?* Forgive me for jesting, but if I wasn't, I'd be cursing at these evil, callous monsters. Keep in mind a vial of this stuff contains 100mg of ALLO. They are charging several thousand dollars for a tenth of a gram. A bottle of pregnenolone that contains three grams costs in the order of ten bucks. I recently bought 100g (3.5 oz) of it in bulk for a whopping $83. There is a special place in hell for these people for profiting off the suffering of new moms who are already under tremendous amounts of stress and likely experiencing sleep deprivation.

They say the treatment needs to be an intravenous infusion because of the poor absorbability or bioavailability of these types of compounds (they are lipids, and it is true to a degree), but if you take them with fat, they absorb enough to have an effect. Sure, you may "waste" some that doesn't get absorbed or is inactivated and excreted by the liver, but hey, it's not like it cost you seven grand per vial! Taking pregnenolone with a meal that contains fat suffices to ensure adequate absorption, but if you want to take it a step further, you can melt a few grams of butter and open the capsule and mix it in. Taken this way, the pregnenolone bypasses the liver and is redirected through the lymphatic system instead.

I remember how profound the change was when my wife and I added pregnenolone to our supplement routine. The package arrived in the late afternoon and, as per my usual over-zealous experimental propensity, instead of titrating the serving slowly as I always advise my clients to do, I took four capsules (200mg) around dinner time. That night, I woke up at 2:30 am and peed out one whole litre of urine, literally. (Why and how I measure how much I pee out at night is a story for another day...)

Whatever it was doing, pregnenolone caused me to wake up before 4 a.m. for the next three days, but I wasn't as cranky as I would have been normally. My sleep normalised after the fourth day and even seemed to improve, as I was sleeping longer than usual and waking up less during the night. I believe the initial water loss was due to the lowering of stress hormones that were causing water retention. What that period taught me is how stressed I actually was, without realising it. You may be the same; I'm convinced the majority of adults out there are. It truly takes experiencing "no-stress" for a while—even for a day or two—to appreciate how neck-deep we are in Stress Mode.

During the next two weeks, my wife and I didn't have any arguments at all. This was uncommon for the period we were in because raising a two-year-old by ourselves with minimal external help meant we were often "on edge". During the second of those weeks, our daughter fell sick like she never had before. A day after a trip to the zoo—with all the usual licking and touching of gross things, followed by putting her hands in her mouth—she developed a fever that lasted almost a week. We did everything we should (such as avoiding a premature trip to the doctor and needless antibiotic and toxic Tylenol prescriptions) and knew the fever was part of the healing process, but near the end, even I was getting worried. As it was the weekend, I planned to take her to the doctor first thing Monday, but by then, thankfully, she was recovering.

Under normal circumstances, we'd be arguing over whether to take her to the doctor, when to use an intervention to lower the temperature, how much of our herbal remedies to give her, and so on. But not this time. No-one raised their voice even once. I was acutely aware of it too, and in disbelief that pregnenolone could do this. I heard similar reports when some of my clients began taking it. People were sleeping through the night for the first in "forever", or were calmer than they had ever been in their adult life. To me, it feels like pregnenolone has a sort of "adaptogenic" effect in the body—as if we utilise it wherever we need it most. It is a most amazing of substances.

As for ALLO, it might not surprise you that some researchers state that it "may have therapeutic potential for treatment of various stress-related diseases including post-traumatic stress disorder (PTSD), depression, alcohol use disorders (AUDs), as well as neurological and psychiatric conditions that are worsened in the presence of stress, such as multiple sclerosis, schizophrenia, and seizure disorders."[9]

Since we know that stress precipitates or worsens virtually every condition, we can expect that most people will benefit from it purely through its anxiolytic and stress-reducing properties. During acute stress, stress hormones elevate while inflammatory signalling increases in the body—but an increase in neuroactive steroids such as ALLO counters this. Chronic stress depletes our protective neurosteroids and causes a decrease in GABA signalling (thus disrupting the equilibrium between the excitatory and inhibitory systems), while stress signalling and inflammatory processes continue to increase.[9] Over time, this imbalance grinds the person down. Adding pregnenolone to this equation can restore ALLO levels and GABA signalling, which can have profound stress-lowering effects.

If all that wasn't enough, pregnenolone has been shown to reduce cravings in alcohol use disorder and cocaine addiction studies.[10][11] These were published in 2022 and 2023, so word will get out soon enough and hopefully much more research will be done. You are ahead of the pack. Since addiction largely stems from trauma and/or stress, and we use various substances to self-medicate in often suboptimal ways, it is promising to see that simply reducing stress signalling in the body and restoring levels of protective neurosteroids can be enough help for a subset of people to overcome their craving for substances that cause harm in the long run (and thus reduce longevity). At that point, if the person has the chance to augment their environment such that substance use cues or triggers are removed, it becomes easier to re-design their life and habits with healthier activities. The key is to reduce the internal stress that prompts the person to reach for their substance of choice because we know that using willpower alone is seldom enough to overcome an addiction.

Finally, while pregnenolone is not available in some countries, progesterone may be available to you over-the-counter, or if not, by doctor's prescription. Keep that in mind, because progesterone can also be converted to ALLO in the body. In fact, it has been shown to reduce cocaine cravings and contribute to improved emotional state by the same research group that studied pregnenolone's effects in alcohol and cocaine use disorders.[12]

Conclusion

There you have it. Actual tools to combat anxiety, depression, sleep problems, and even addiction. No fluff and no need to meditate an hour a day and visualise unicorns showering you with rainbows of loving serenity. Unless you want to, of course.

I can't remove the psychological stressors from your life. Only you can. We also need to accept that certain stressors cannot be fully eliminated. But that doesn't mean we need to suffer through them or blunt our response with sedative drugs. It took me decades of suffering and self-medication to learn that, hence I'm glad I can help others shortcut this process. The tools I've laid out here are simple, but they are your proverbial hammer, screwdriver, and measuring tape. You can build a lot of projects with them, and while you are free to explore and experiment with the hundreds of options out there, keep these in your back pocket as they can make all the difference. And remember, just because you have ways to reduce stress, does not mean you should add more of it in your life—that's the opposite of a longevity strategy!

7. Give Your Gut Some Love

The more I learn about the various ways in which gut dysfunction contributes to physical and psychological health problems, the more I'm amazed at the wisdom of Hippocrates—whose most famous quote is that "all disease begins in the gut". If the body is a wheel, the gastrointestinal (GI) tract is the axis; should it malfunction, every spoke can be affected. Virtually every client I work with either has an overt gut issue (gas, indigestion, bloating, constipation), or we uncover hidden GI imbalances upon deeper investigation. This is the case even when their main health complaint seems to be completely unrelated to the gut (e.g., fatigue, brain fog, skin issues, or weight gain). Thankfully, because the gastrointestinal tract affects every other system in the body directly or indirectly, improving its functioning usually confers wide-ranging benefits.

My first-hand experience of how gut pathogens can wreck your health without you even knowing it was in 2019. As part of my Functional Diagnostic Nutrition (FDN) training, I needed to run an advanced hormone panel on myself. This is a collect-at-home test—called the DUTCH, which stands for "dried urine test for comprehensive hormones"—that maps out your sex hormones (androgens, estrogens and their metabolites), adrenal hormones (including cortisol and how it rises and falls in a 24-hour period), and various organic acids that give insight into aspects of the metabolism such as neurotransmitters, B-vitamins, and oxidative stress. I was one of the first FDN trainees to get to run it, as it was going to replace the previous salivary cortisol test, and boy was I pumped to see the results. But when I did, my excitement turned to surprise, then quickly to disbelief.

There I was expecting my FDN course mentor to be floored by my near-optimal hormone levels and to say something like, "You got this, Chris. You don't need my help!" or "Teach me your secrets, oh Great One with the perfect lab results!" Yet the picture was very different. My androgen levels were *tanked*, with some markers *below* the bottom of the range for my age group. Cortisol was sky high, and my protective hormones (such as DHEA) were near the bottom of the range. When I said I was in disbelief, I meant it. As soon as we finished the session with my mentor, I called the lab to enquire whether their state-of-the-art equipment needed to be calibrated… Really. The lady on the phone was polite, but probably thought she was talking with a loop-the-loop.

I was travelling that week and couldn't get immediate testing done, so my next move was to run out in search of health stores. A few hours later, I was popping capsules with horny goat weed, tribulus terrestris, nettle leaf, and adaptogens like ginseng—all supposed to help with hormonal function and adrenal balance. (Please note, this is not something I ever advocate others to do; I always recommend starting supplements one at a time and gradually titrating each one so you can identify reactions quickly. But my risk tolerance is high and I never really react to anything. Plus, I like to "stress test" compounds before I recommend them to others.)

When I flew home a few days later, I ran blood tests to corroborate the findings of the DUTCH test. My total testosterone was 619 ng/dl, which by today's standards may not be low, but I was certainly feeling weak. That was more than a month after I had collected the DUTCH test sample and after a few days on the herbal protocol, so it's difficult to say how low it was at the time of test collection. It was only in hindsight that I realised how "off" things had been. My libido was certainly not at its normal levels. It felt like I was forcing myself to exercise. I was going to bed as early as 9 p.m., only to wake up in the middle of the night and struggle to fall back asleep. Not to mention the ungodly amounts of coffee I was pouring down my neck.

My Oura ring (a biometric tracking device I was using) rarely reported that my sleep and recovery were even close to optimal, which, until the hormone test, had me questioning how well it was even working. (I didn't call the company to blame their algorithms or technology, in this case.) Our diet was great, I was on a cocktail of supplements, and was devouring the most prominent biohackers' best content—how I could I have *any* imbalances? I wasn't the first nor the last to delude myself that I was perfectly healthy—many men suffer from this, to their eventual detriment. This experience humbled me and I'm grateful I learned the lesson relatively early.

My FDN mentor told me that parasites or heavy metals could have caused my low hormones, so I promptly ordered the comprehensive GI-MAP (GI Microbial Assay Plus) stool test and sent my first hair sample off for trace mineral and toxic metal analysis. The excitement of running new labs took my mind off how lousy I felt.

As soon as I collected the stool sample, I tucked into several cloves of fresh garlic as an opening salvo; the preemptively purchased gut cleansing reinforcements were on their way, but I wasn't wasting any time. This was war, and a lot of tiny one-celled bastards were about to be meet their maker. A coalition of additional anti-bacterial herbs from my local health store were soon deployed to the battlefield. Those poor unsuspecting microbes didn't even see it coming. It was pandemonium. Throughout that first night, the cannons were firing relentlessly, if you catch my drift. The seemingly endless gas and bloating were uncomfortable, but as I said, I'm not overly sensitive. Please do not try this at home! It can be extremely unpleasant (or even dangerous) to kill tons of pathogens quickly without a strategy on how to deal with the die-off.

As I had also stopped drinking coffee to give my adrenals a break, the next few days were spent either sleeping or camped out on the couch. As the battle was raging on, my wife was quite worried; being so lethargic was completely out of character for me. But soon enough, I was feeling better.

Less than a month later, the GI-MAP results showed I had *Giardia* and the protozoa *Blastocystis hominis*, alongside an overgrowth of the yeast *Candida* and several bacterial species that can be harmful if not kept in check. Phew. That explained it.

I believe my experiments with raw meat may have exposed me to the pathogens. At the time, I would lay on an acupressure mat on the floor after lunch as a pleasant way to relax and take pressure off my lower back. One day I fell asleep on it, so instead of the usual twenty minutes, I had spent closer to an hour on the cold floor. My guess is my body temperature dropped for long enough to allow the harmful organisms to take hold. I experienced low-grade fever for two or three days after that, but no other symptoms of "infection", so I thought little of it. Reaching my state of diminished health was a slow progression that was difficult to pinpoint to a specific event.

Though most likely self-inflicted, this period spurred me on to learn how to address gut problems comprehensively and now allows me to have empathy for others who are suffering in a similar way. These days, I can almost "sense" when a prospective client has some low-grade chronic gut dysbiosis that doesn't cause overt GI symptoms but is otherwise messing with their health.

I'm certain many people are currently living with dysfunction that originated in a similar way to mine. Their immune system, gut lining, or gut microbiota may have been compromised by any combination of factors—stress, illness, or toxins from food, bacteria, or the environment—which allows organisms that are normally not problematic to overgrow, or less often, for pathogens to colonise the intestine. When my clients choose to run stool pathogen tests, it's rare that we see an overt pathogen such as *Salmonella*, *Cryptosporidium*, or *Clostridium difficile*. More often, there is an overgrowth of so-called "opportunistic" bacteria that the normal microbiota has failed to keep at bay. Some of these opportunists are known to trigger inflammatory or autoimmune processes that may contribute to dysfunction in the gut and beyond.

Endotoxin: the ubiquitous inflammatory trigger

Here is what most people don't know: You don't need to be "colonised" or infected to experience problems from the bacteria in your gut. There are certain types called *gram-negative* bacteria that have millions of fragments in their cell walls that are highly inflammatory. These bacterial cell wall fragments are called *endotoxin,* or LPS (*lipopolysaccharide*). Most of the endotoxin-producing bacteria live in the gut, though some species also live on our skin and gums. Certain cells in the body have receptors that recognise these endotoxin particles and, when activated by them, the cells initiate a strong inflammatory response. And no-one is exempt—we all have these types of bacteria in our gastrointestinal tracts.

> Gram-negative bacteria, containing endotoxin, are found at very high levels in the mammalian gut (mainly lower intestine)[1]

While certain pathogenic gram-negative species can cause overt gastrointestinal, urinary, or respiratory problems, and even meningitis, others are considered to be members of our regular microbiota or to only become problematic when allowed to overgrow. As it happens, we're highly sensitive to the endotoxin these bacteria produce:

> Humans are orders of magnitude more sensitive to endotoxin than other mammals, such as mice.[1]

What's interesting is that "the toxicity of endotoxin is due to the host's inflammatory over-reaction to it, rather than an intrinsic toxicity to animal cells."[1] Endotoxin comprises lipid (*lipo-*) and carbohydrate (*saccharide*) molecules, which are not inherently dangerous. It is the *perception* by the body that it is under attack by a pathogen that causes it to create an inflammatory cascade intended to neutralise the would-be attacker. It is this inflammatory overreaction, especially when chronically activated (as it is in many people), that wreaks havoc on our health.

Just how sensitive are we to endotoxin? In "experimental endotoxemia", when human volunteers are injected with one nanogram of endotoxin per kilogram of body mass—that's one tenth of a microgram for a 100kg person, which is 0.0001 milligrams—they experience increased sickness behaviour (fatigue, headache, muscle pain, shivering) and decreased motivation (alertness, energy, focus, pep, social interest) within a couple of hours, along with increased inflammation. The things we do for money, eh?

Researchers have also shown that experimental endotoxemia induces insulin resistance in humans, adding another piece to the puzzle of this issue that—as you now know—is much more nuanced than the mainstream "too many carbs and sugar" narrative.[2] In its most serious manifestation, high levels of endotoxin in the blood can cause a "cytokine storm", septic shock, and death. But it's the chronic low levels of endotoxin, which are a source of low-grade inflammation, that predispose us to accelerated ageing and disease. Similar to the dysregulated stress response, this is another example of how a beautifully designed survival mechanism becomes harmful when continually activated.

Hence, as you may expect, blood endotoxin levels are elevated in various health conditions, including obesity, insulin resistance, diabetes, non-alcoholic fatty liver disease (NAFLD), chronic infection, and cardiovascular and neurodegenerative disease.[1][3-7] A person with atherosclerosis may have three times the amount of those in a healthy human,[1] and researchers who found endotoxin in human atherosclerotic plaque (it was probably that evil cholesterol that put it there) stated that:

> ...in patients at risk of cardiovascular events circulating LPS [endotoxin] concentration independently predicted myocardial infarction, stroke and cardiovascular death during a follow-up of about 3 years[4]

As for the implications of increased endotoxin and ageing and loss of function, researchers have reported:

> In healthy older individuals higher levels of the lipopolysaccharide binding protein (LBP) were associated with higher inflammation and worse physical function.[8]

When gram-negative bacteria complete their lifecycle and die, the cells rupture and spill their contents into the gastrointestinal tract. This is where the harmful effects of endotoxin particles begin by increasing gut "permeability".[9][10] Also known as "leaky gut", this is a state where the gaps between your intestinal cells increase such that they allow undigested bits of food and toxins (bacterial, chemical, etc.) to enter the bloodstream (these would not normally be allowed in by the intestinal cells).

Once endotoxin is in your blood, it can cause brain inflammation through the inflammatory responses it triggers in the periphery or by entering the brain. Over time, this can lead to neurodegeneration. Hence, it's not surprising that blood endotoxin levels in Alzheimer's disease can be as much as six times higher than those in healthy people. In rodent experiments (and remember humans are far more sensitive to endotoxin), a single injection with endotoxin results in activation of immune cells in the brain that lasts for at least 12 months, whereas chronic doses cause more rapid neurodegeneration akin to that in Parkinson's or Alzheimer's disease. Those poor lab animals just cannot catch a break.

All that was to say: you need to take endotoxin seriously. Since we all harbour species that produce it, we need to stay on top of them like a diligent gardener ensures the weeds don't overgrow and pests don't ruin the crops.

Let's talk about solutions. The overarching goal is probably clear: You need to keep endotoxin levels as low as possible and make sure your gut is in excellent working order because increased intestinal permeability is the gateway through which endotoxin passes to enter the bloodstream. You also need to keep your liver in good nick because it degrades and clears most of the endotoxin in the blood—a topic we'll cover in depth in the next volume of this series.

Longevity tip: Don't feed endotoxin-producing bacteria too much!

Now, I risk being burned at the stake for this blasphemy, but let me tell you outright: eating a boatload of fibre, more specifically the *soluble* kind, is *not* necessarily beneficial for your gut—especially if you have no idea if you have an overgrowth of gram-negative bacteria (which a stool test can shed light on). The fact is, every time you consume resistant starches and fibre, you're indiscriminately feeding all species that can ferment these indigestible-for-us materials. That includes the endotoxin-producing species.

Since we know endotoxin can increase leaky gut and cause damaging inflammation once in our bloodstream, my personal longevity strategy is to limit as much as possible the biggest sources of fibre and resistant starches—namely seeds of all kinds including beans, grains, lentils, and nuts. It may go against the mainstream "grain", where fibre is promoted as the incredible cholesterol-lowering, cancer-risk reducing, gut bacteria-feeding gift from plants that we all ought to eat more of, but you should understand by now why I'm comfortable with my choices.

Please note that unlike PUFAs, where "as little as humanly possible without going crazy" is probably the ideal amount, having fibre here and there is not going to be a problem for most people, unless they have extreme gut dysfunction. So I wouldn't worry about the fibre in fruit or the occasional indulgence—I just wouldn't go out of my way to add extra resistant starch from supplements like inulin or green bananas or by eating cold potatoes or grains (like some cooky characters are recommending).

If you are healthy with a well-functioning gut lining, feeding the gram-negative bacteria extra fibre may not pose a visible problem. However, if you have some degree of intestinal permeability, your baseline inflammation may rise but it would be near-impossible to "feel" or detect it without lab testing. Allowing the opportunistic bacteria to proliferate is, in many ways, a ticking time-bomb. The more-benign organisms in the gut will keep them at bay, but if your microbiota or gut lining are compromised for any reason (unhealthy lifestyle, antibiotics, drugs, immune system dysregulation, etc.), you could be in trouble.

Now, you may be worried that too little fibre will constipate you, and that is understandable, given the conditioning we're subjected to. However, you need to understand that virtually all the studies portraying fibre as beneficial are epidemiological in nature—i.e., few actual experiments were conducted—and only show *associations* between (usually self-reported) food intake and health outcomes. No *causality* is demonstrated. This type of research is plagued by poor recall of the survey participants and myriad confounding variables. One example is the "healthy user bias", where participants may engage in multiple "healthy" behaviours, which makes it difficult to ascertain that, for example, it was the high fibre intake that reduced their "risk" (which is a misnomer) of colorectal cancer and not the fact they eat higher quality food, avoid processed products, and drink less alcohol.

The authors give credence to their papers by stating that "higher intake of X reduces the risk of Y", where they should state that "higher intake of X is *associated* with a reduced *incidence* of Y (in this small sample of the population)". Sleight of hand like this, especially when magnified by the mainstream media, can readily shape the perceptions of the public.

An actual interventional study published in the *World Journal of Gastroenterology*, tellingly titled "Stopping or reducing dietary fiber intake reduces constipation and its associated symptoms", concluded this:

> Idiopathic constipation and its associated symptoms can be effectively reduced by stopping or even lowering the intake of dietary fiber.[11]

Sixty-three people with idiopathic (of unknown origin) constipation participated in the study. Of them, 41 were on a no-fibre diet for six months. Not only did their stool frequency increase from an average of 3.75 days to once per day, their symptoms of bloating and straining to pass stools were completely resolved.

> Patients who stopped or reduced dietary fiber had significant improvement in their symptoms while those who continued on a high fiber diet had no change. Of those who stopped fiber completely, the bowel frequency increased from one motion in 3.75 d ($\pm$ 1.59 d) to one motion in 1.0 d [...]; those with reduced fiber intake had increased bowel frequency from a mean of one motion per 4.19 d ($\pm$ 2.09 d) to one motion per 1.9 d ($\pm$ 1.21 d) on a reduced fiber diet [...]; those who remained on a high fiber diet continued to have a mean of one motion per 6.83 d ($\pm$ 1.03 d) before and after consultation. For no fiber, reduced fiber and high fiber groups, respectively, symptoms of bloating were present in 0%, 31.3% and 100% [...] and straining to pass stools occurred in 0%, 43.8% and 100% [...].[11]

It's bewildering that none of the high-fibre diet participants saw any improvement during the six months. You'd think the placebo effect of participating in a study would have played at least a minor role. I guess shovelling more indigestible crap down an already congested tube isn't magically going to "unblock" it. Maybe they should have tried using a plunger…

Longevity tip: "Block" the inflammatory cascade caused by endotoxin with pregnenolone

You could probably tell from the previous chapter that I'm pretty excited about pregnenolone. As it turns out, it and its metabolite allopregnanolone (ALLO) can suppress the inflammatory response caused by endotoxin via interplay with the receptors that "sense" it. Without getting too technical, endotoxin is recognised by receptors called TLR (toll-like receptors) and when it attaches to them, the inflammatory cascade is triggered. This can happen in the periphery but also in the brain, which is highly undesirable, as the resultant neuroinflammation can damage brain cells. Pregnenolone and ALLO inhibit this pro-inflammatory activation at the receptor level, hence their anti-inflammatory and neuroprotective properties.[12][13] Pretty nifty, isn't it? To me, pregnenolone is the gift that keeps on giving. If I woke up one day to find out it had washed my car and thrown out the diaper bin, I wouldn't be too surprised.

Longevity tip: "Mop up" endotoxin in your gut with activated charcoal

For many people, the primary benefits of intermittent or water fasting stem from giving their gut a break.[14] A prolonged period without inflammatory foods and starches and fibres that feed endotoxin-producing bacteria allows the gut lining to repair itself, and thus for intestinal permeability to be reduced. This results in less endotoxin entering the bloodstream when the person eats their next meal, which creates a positive feedforward cycle. Therein lies the solution to lowering inflammation and improving gut health without the added stress and collateral damage of fasting: reduce fermentable substrates, remove the inflammatory and processed junk, and add nutrient-rich and easily digestible foods. It is so simple that you could teach it to a doct…never mind.

To take it a step further, use 1-3g of activated charcoal two-to-three times per week to add another layer of protection. Activated charcoal binds toxins in the gut—which prevents them from slipping into the bloodstream—and is an almost effortless way to get one benefit of fasting (i.e., a reduction in endotoxin) without starving yourself. Because it is a binder, the best way to take it is on an empty stomach (with a glass of water) between meals; ideally two hours before and after food and supplements. Since such gaps aren't always possible, you don't need to strive for perfection. For many people, it is easiest to take it last thing at night.

Keep in mind that if you feel noticeably better after taking activated charcoal, it is firm evidence that you may have an overgrowth in the gut that needs to be "culled", which, as you shall see, is something I consider an essential part to a well-rounded longevity plan.

Longevity tip: "Mow the lawn" once in a while

After the overview of endotoxin, you understand why—contrary to "expert" opinion—shoving all manner of indigestible plant fibres down our gullet is not exactly an optimal strategy for long-term health. In fact, I am of the ardent belief that many of us have health issues precisely (or at least in part) due to an overgrowth of the so-called opportunistic or "dysbiotic" bacteria—many of which are endotoxin-producing. So rather than feeding them, especially when we don't know the lay of the land, the occasional gentle herbal cleanse is a more prudent approach. I personally do this at least twice a year since my whole run-in with *Giardia* and *Blasto* and what-have-you.

There are many ways to skin this cat, and while I'll give you basic guidelines here, keep in mind this information is for educational purposes only. I would urge you to seek professional help if you have an evident gut issue, because I've seen folks make things a lot worse for themselves with random trial and error—please exercise extreme caution. Also, while I go pretty heavy with my personal gut cleansing protocols, it is always best to follow the "low-and-slow" approach, especially if it is your first gut cleanse. By that, I mean always start one supplement at a time and use the lowest possible serving size, then increase it gradually while monitoring yourself for reactions, which I'll explain shortly. You can check the online appendix for examples of products I use.

My go to is to use liquid olive leaf extract as a gentle "opening act". If there is indeed an overgrowth and increased intestinal permeability, the last thing you want is to start killing organisms left and right. Some of the dead matter (including endotoxin) could make it into your bloodstream and cause an immune reaction that may be uncomfortable and even damaging.

Starting with 1 drop on an empty stomach, 15-30 minutes before meals, I'd gradually increase it to three times per day. If comfortable, I slowly increase the number of drops at each serving until I'm on ten drops, three times per day. As this is getting ramped up, I would add 500-1000mg of activated charcoal every day or second day to "mop up" any die-off, as explained earlier. An optional and usually beneficial practice is to add a probiotic during the protocol, such as a *lactobacillus/bifidobacterium* mix (about 50 billion CFUs), or my current favourite, the spore-forming *bacillus coagulans*, which can be taken with food.

If no "die-off" reactions such as headache, fever, chills, lethargy, muscle pain, or anxiety have been felt until now, I would feel comfortable adding a drop of oregano oil with each serving and increasing it to five-to-ten drops. Since oregano oil is very strong (you'll understand what I mean if you try it), most people need to dilute it in a little juice or other liquid such as olive oil.

Die-off symptoms (also known as a *Herxheimer* reaction) indicate that the protocol is working; however, because they are uncomfortable, we want to keep them at a low level. To do this, we taper back on the herbals for a day or two (e.g., use half the number of drops) and increase fluid intake and binders such as activated charcoal to deal with excess toxins and bacterial metabolites in the gut.

Further additions to the above can include fresh garlic (crushed, chopped, then left to stand for 10 minutes before ingesting) or garlic extract (allicin), as they have broad spectrum anti-bacterial properties. You may also add two or three daily servings of grapefruit seed extract for its potent anti-yeast (e.g., *Candida*) properties (always take it on an empty stomach and never mix with other supplements).

My personal indication that the protocol has done its job is if I can maintain it at the maximum drops of olive leaf extract and oregano oil (and any other additions) for 10-20 days without feeling any different (i.e., no die-reactions). This usually means there are no heavy overgrowths (or you're dealing with the die-off well). After doing this once, the maintenance cleanse can be shorter—a week or two. My preference is to do it twice a year in the spring and autumn, with the occasional three-to-four day mini-cleanse when I feel the need. As you do this more often, you'll "tune in" to your gut and digestion more, and they'll tell you if something is off.

To reiterate, this is a basic way to "mow the lawn" that will reduce overgrowths, but it won't necessarily address more serious dysbiosis and infections such as parasites, worms, or specific pathogenic bacteria. Different organisms require different strategies and protocol lengths, so I once again urge you to seek professional help if you feel you have a gut issue that is deep-seated. In these instances, testing for pathogens with a comprehensive stool test is valuable because it can save you the fruitless trial-and-error that sometimes makes things worse.

Conclusion

In a nutshell, this is the simple and effective strategy to keep your gut healthy long-term: Remove inflammatory foods and junk from your diet. Reduce endotoxin-producing bacteria numbers and keep them low by not feeding them too much fermentable plant matter. Bind toxins in the gut with activated charcoal now and then. Use pregnenolone to block the inflammatory cascade, in case some endotoxin makes it into the bloodstream.

As mentioned, in the next volume of this series, I'll show you further ways to overhaul your gastrointestinal and digestive system, which includes the liver and gallbladder—two organs that are given very little attention. Until then, see overleaf how you can accelerate your journey to optimal health and longevity…

Accelerate Your Journey to Optimal Health

I hope you found the information in this volume valuable. It has taken me years and thousands of hours of research and experimentation to get here, and I'm glad to pass on the knowledge so others may reap the benefits. As a reminder, the online appendix contains links to products I use that were mentioned in the book: **HowToActuallyLiveLonger.com/vol-1**

Though I already know the topics and strategies that will be discussed the next two volumes (at least) and use them in my work with clients, the time-consuming nature of the research, writing, editing, and publishing process means there will be a significant time-delay between each volume.

In the meantime, if you want personalised help with optimising your metabolic function or addressing a chronic issue, I invite you to visit my website and request a free introductory call: **https://HowToActuallyLiveLonger.com/**

We'll use this session to understand your health goals and see if you are fit for my health optimisation and longevity program. If you are, we will take you to the next level(s) using state-of-the-art functional lab testing and protocols that address nutrition, supplementation, gut health, detoxification, sleep, stress reduction, inflammation, oxidative stress, and other important areas.

Scan the QR code to visit the website:

About the author

Christian Yordanov is a health author and Functional Diagnostic Nutrition Practitioner. He has worked with clients with severe gastrointestinal ailments, toxicity, and debilitating chronic fatigue. He has helped people with autoimmune and neurological conditions, skin disorders, hypothyroidism, insomnia, depression, autism, obesity, and other metabolic problems. The clients he serves are busy parents, professionals, executives, and entrepreneurs.

In his clinical work, Christian uses functional lab testing to identify hidden metabolic and health imbalances, and teaches clients how to use diet, supplementation, detoxification, stress reduction, sleep optimisation, and other strategies to address their chronic health issues and transform their lives for the better.

Learn more about his health optimisation and longevity program at: **https://HowToActuallyLiveLonger.com/**

References

Introduction

1. Kumar P, Liu C, Hsu JW, Chacko S, Minard C, Jahoor F, Sekhar RV. Glycine and N-acetylcysteine (GlyNAC) supplementation in older adults improves glutathione deficiency, oxidative stress, mitochondrial dysfunction, inflammation, insulin resistance, endothelial dysfunction, genotoxicity, muscle strength, and cognition: Results of a pilot clinical trial. Clin Transl Med. 2021 Mar;11(3):e372. doi: 10.1002/ctm2.372. PMID: 33783984; PMCID: PMC8002905.

Chapter 1

1. López-Otín C, Blasco MA, Partridge L, Serrano M, Kroemer G. The hallmarks of aging. Cell. 2013 Jun 6;153(6):1194-217. doi: 10.1016/j.cell.2013.05.039. PMID: 23746838; PMCID: PMC3836174.

2. Cesari M, Penninx BW, Pahor M, Lauretani F, Corsi AM, Rhys Williams G, Guralnik JM, Ferrucci L. Inflammatory markers and physical performance in older persons: the InCHIANTI study. J Gerontol A Biol Sci Med Sci. 2004 Mar;59(3):242-8. doi: 10.1093/gerona/59.3.m242. PMID: 15031308.

3. Brinkley TE, Leng X, Miller ME, Kitzman DW, Pahor M, Berry MJ, Marsh AP, Kritchevsky SB, Nicklas BJ. Chronic inflammation is associated with low physical function in older adults across multiple comorbidities. J Gerontol A Biol Sci Med Sci. 2009 Apr;64(4):455-61. doi: 10.1093/gerona/gln038. Epub 2009 Feb 4. PMID: 19196644; PMCID: PMC2657165.

4. Schaap LA, Pluijm SM, Deeg DJ, Visser M. Inflammatory markers and loss of muscle mass (sarcopenia) and strength. Am J Med. 2006 Jun;119(6):526.e9-17. doi: 10.1016/j.amjmed.2005.10.049. PMID: 16750969.

5. Sousa AC, Zunzunegui MV, Li A, Phillips SP, Guralnik JM, Guerra

RO. Association between C-reactive protein and physical performance in older populations: results from the International Mobility in Aging Study (IMIAS). Age Ageing. 2016 Mar;45(2):274-80. doi: 10.1093/ageing/afv202. Epub 2016 Jan 28. PMID: 26822196.

6.   Mishra SK, Balendra V, Esposto J, Obaid AA, Maccioni RB, Jha NK, Perry G, Moustafa M, Al-Shehri M, Singh MP, Khan AA, Vamanu E, Singh SK. Therapeutic Antiaging Strategies. Biomedicines. 2022 Oct 8;10(10):2515. doi: 10.3390/biomedicines10102515. PMID: 36289777; PMCID: PMC9599338.

7.   Kumar P, Liu C, Hsu JW, Chacko S, Minard C, Jahoor F, Sekhar RV. Glycine and N-acetylcysteine (GlyNAC) supplementation in older adults improves glutathione deficiency, oxidative stress, mitochondrial dysfunction, inflammation, insulin resistance, endothelial dysfunction, genotoxicity, muscle strength, and cognition: Results of a pilot clinical trial. Clin Transl Med. 2021 Mar;11(3):e372. doi: 10.1002/ctm2.372. PMID: 33783984; PMCID: PMC8002905.

8.   Chi GC, Fitzpatrick AL, Sharma M, Jenny NS, Lopez OL, DeKosky ST. Inflammatory Biomarkers Predict Domain-Specific Cognitive Decline in Older Adults. J Gerontol A Biol Sci Med Sci. 2017 Jun 1;72(6):796-803. doi: 10.1093/gerona/glw155. PMID: 27522059; PMCID: PMC5861845.

9.   Black CN, Bot M, Scheffer PG, Cuijpers P, Penninx BW. Is depression associated with increased oxidative stress? A systematic review and meta-analysis. Psychoneuroendocrinology. 2015 Jan;51:164-75. doi: 10.1016/j.psyneuen.2014.09.025. Epub 2014 Oct 2. PMID: 25462890.

10.   McEwen BS. Protection and damage from acute and chronic stress: allostasis and allostatic overload and relevance to the pathophysiology of psychiatric disorders. Ann N Y Acad Sci. 2004 Dec;1032:1-7. doi: 10.1196/annals.1314.001. PMID: 15677391.

11.   Vogelzangs N, Beekman AT, Milaneschi Y, Bandinelli S, Ferrucci L, Penninx BW. Urinary cortisol and six-year risk of all-cause and cardiovascular mortality. J Clin Endocrinol Metab. 2010 Nov;95(11):4959-64. doi: 10.1210/jc.2010-0192. Epub 2010 Aug 25. PMID: 20739384; PMCID: PMC2968721.

12.   Sapse AT. Cortisol, high cortisol diseases and anti-cortisol therapy. Psychoneuroendocrinology. 1997;22 Suppl 1:S3-10. doi: 10.1016/s0306-4530(97)00024-3. PMID: 9264141.

13.   Nashel DJ. Is atherosclerosis a complication of long-term corticosteroid treatment? Am J Med. 1986 May;80(5):925-9. doi: 10.1016/0002-9343(86)90639-x. PMID: 3518440.

14.   Kenna, H.A., Poon, A.W., de los Angeles, C.P. and Koran, L.M. (2011), Psychiatric complications of treatment with corticosteroids:

176

Review with case report. Psychiatry and Clinical Neurosciences, 65: 549-560. https://doi.org/10.1111/j.1440-1819.2011.02260.x

15. Sacks O, Shulman M. Steroid dementia: an overlooked diagnosis? Neurology. 2005 Feb 22;64(4):707-9. doi: 10.1212/01.WNL.0000151977.18440.C3. PMID: 15728296.

16. Wright CE, Kunz-Ebrecht SR, Iliffe S, Foese O, Steptoe A. Physiological correlates of cognitive functioning in an elderly population. Psychoneuroendocrinology. 2005 Oct;30(9):826-38. doi: 10.1016/j.psyneuen.2005.04.001. PMID: 15975730.

17. Noordam, Raymond; Gunn, David A.; Tomlin, Cyrena C.; Rozing, Maarten P.; Maier, Andrea B.; Slagboom, P. Eline; Westendorp, Rudi G.J.; van Heemst, Diana; de Craen, Anton J.M. (2012). Cortisol serum levels in familial longevity and perceived age: The Leiden Longevity Study. Psychoneuroendocrinology, 37(10), 1669–1675. doi:10.1016/j.psyneuen.2012.02.013

18. Christensen K, Thinggaard M, McGue M, Rexbye H, Hjelmborg J v B, Aviv A et al. Perceived age as clinically useful biomarker of ageing: cohort study BMJ 2009; 339 :b5262 doi:10.1136/bmj.b5262

19. Zannas AS. Epigenetics as a key link between psychosocial stress and aging: concepts, evidence, mechanisms. Dialogues Clin Neurosci. 2019 Dec;21(4):389-396. doi: 10.31887/DCNS.2019.21.4/azannas. PMID: 31949406; PMCID: PMC6952744.

Chapter 2

1. Péter S, Friedel A, Roos FF, Wyss A, Eggersdorfer M, Hoffmann K, Weber P. A Systematic Review of Global Alpha-Tocopherol Status as Assessed by Nutritional Intake Levels and Blood Serum Concentrations. Int J Vitam Nutr Res. 2015 Dec;85(5-6):261-281. doi: 10.1024/0300-9831/a000281. Epub 2016 Jul 14. PMID: 27414419.

2. Guyenet SJ, Carlson SE. Increase in adipose tissue linoleic acid of US adults in the last half century. Adv Nutr 2015;6:660–4.doi:10.3945/an.115.009944

3. McBurney MI, Yu EA, Ciappio ED, Bird JK, Eggersdorfer M, Mehta S. Suboptimal Serum α-Tocopherol Concentrations Observed among Younger Adults and Those Depending Exclusively upon Food Sources, NHANES 2003-20061-3. PLoS One. 2015 Aug 19;10(8):e0135510. doi: 10.1371/journal.pone.0135510. PMID: 26287975; PMCID: PMC4546010.

4. Shaikh SR, Edidin M. Immunosuppressive effects of polyunsaturat-

ed fatty acids on antigen presentation by human leukocyte antigen class I molecules. J Lipid Res. 2007 Jan;48(1):127-38. doi: 10.1194/jlr.M600365-JLR200. Epub 2006 Oct 30. PMID: 17074926.

5. McHugh MI, Wilkinson R, Elliott RW, Field EJ, Dewar P, Hall RR, Taylor RM, Uldall PR. Immunosuppression with polyunsaturated fatty acids in renal transplantation. Transplantation. 1977 Oct;24(4):263-7. doi: 10.1097/00007890-197710000-00005. PMID: 335584.

6. Mamounis, Kyle. (2017). The Dangers of Fat Metabolism and PUFA: Why You Don't Want to be a Fat Burner. Journal of Evolution and Health. 2. 10.15310/2334-3591.1048.

7. Chopra IJ, Huang TS, Beredo A, Solomon DH, Chua Teco GN, Mead JF. Evidence for an inhibitor of extrathyroidal conversion of thyroxine to 3,5,3'-triiodothyronine in sera of patients with nonthyroidal illnesses. J Clin Endocrinol Metab 1985;60:666–72. doi:10.1210/jcem-60-4-666.

8. Tabachnick M, Korcek L. Effect of long-chain fatty acids on the binding of thyroxine and triiodothyronine to human thyroxine-binding globulin. Biochim Biophys Acta - Gen Subj 1986;881:292–6. doi:10.1016/0304-4165(86)90016-4.

9. Wiersinga WM, Chopra IJ, Teco GN. Inhibition of nuclear T3 binding by fatty acids. Metabolism. 1988 Oct;37(10):996-1002. doi: 10.1016/0026-0495(88)90159-x. PMID: 3173114.

10. Giroud S, Frare C, Strijkstra A, Boerema A, Arnold W, Ruf T. Membrane phospholipid fatty acid composition regulates cardiac SERCA activity in a hibernator, the Syrian hamster (Mesocricetus auratus). PLoS One. 2013 May 1;8(5):e63111. doi: 10.1371/journal.pone.0063111. PMID: 23650545; PMCID: PMC3641109.

11. Negre-Salvayre A, Auge N, Ayala V, Basaga H, Boada J, Brenke R, Chapple S, Cohen G, Feher J, Grune T, Lengyel G, Mann GE, Pamplona R, Poli G, Portero-Otin M, Riahi Y, Salvayre R, Sasson S, Serrano J, Shamni O, Siems W, Siow RC, Wiswedel I, Zarkovic K, Zarkovic N. Pathological aspects of lipid peroxidation. Free Radic Res. 2010 Oct;44(10):1125-71. doi: 10.3109/10715762.2010.498478. PMID: 20836660.

12. Romano A, Serviddio G, Calcagnini S, Villani R, Giudetti AM, Cassano T, Gaetani S. Linking lipid peroxidation and neuropsychiatric disorders: focus on 4-hydroxy-2-nonenal. Free Radic Biol Med. 2017 Oct;111:281-293. doi: 10.1016/j.freeradbiomed.2016.12.046. Epub 2017 Jan 4. PMID: 28063940.

13. Di Domenico F, Tramutola A, Butterfield DA. Role of 4-hydroxy-

2-nonenal (HNE) in the pathogenesis of alzheimer disease and other selected age-related neurodegenerative disorders. Free Radic Biol Med. 2017 Oct;111:253-261. doi: 10.1016/j.freeradbiomed.2016.10.490. Epub 2016 Oct 24. PMID: 27789292.

14. Gilani A, Agostinucci K, Hossain S, Pascale JV, Garcia V, Adebesin AM, Falck JR, Schwartzman ML. 20-HETE interferes with insulin signaling and contributes to obesity-driven insulin resistance. Prostaglandins Other Lipid Mediat. 2021 Feb; 152:106485. doi: 10.1016/j.prostaglandins.2020.106485. Epub 2020 Oct 1. PMID: 33011364; PMCID: PMC7855891.

15. Ward NC, Hodgson JM, Puddey IB, Beilin LJ, Croft KD. 20-Hydroxyeicosatetraenoic acid is not associated with circulating insulin in lean to overweight humans. Diabetes Res Clin Pract. 2006 Nov;74(2):197-200. doi: 10.1016/j.diabres.2006.04.001. Epub 2006 May 19. PMID: 16713008.

16. Seppanen, C.M. and Csallany, A.S. (2006), The effect of intermittent and continuous heating of soybean oil at frying temperature on the formation of 4-hydroxy-2-trans-nonenal and other α-, β-unsaturated hydroxyaldehydes. J Amer Oil Chem Soc, 83: 121-127. https://doi.org/10.1007/s11746-006-1184-0

17. Turpeinen AM, Basu S, Mutanen M. A high linoleic acid diet increases oxidative stress in vivo and affects nitric oxde metabolism in humans. Prostaglandins Leukot Essent Fatty Acids. 1998 Sep;59(3):229-33. doi: 10.1016/s0952-3278(98)90067-9. PMID: 9844997.

18. https://www.heart.org/en/healthy-living/healthy-eating/eat-smart/fats/polyunsaturated-fats; Accessed 14 December 2023.

19. Teicholz N. A short history of saturated fat: the making and un-making of a scientific consensus. Curr Opin Endocrinol Diabetes Obes. 2023 Feb 1;30(1):65-71. doi: 10.1097/MED.0000000000000791. Epub 2022 Dec 8. PMID: 36477384; PMCID: PMC9794145.

20. DiNicolantonio JJ, O'Keefe JH. Omega-6 vegetable oils as a driver of coronary heart disease: the oxidized linoleic acid hypothesis. Open Heart. 2018 Sep 26;5(2):e000898. doi: 10.1136/openhrt-2018-000898. PMID: 30364556; PMCID: PMC6196963.

21. Yam D, Eliraz A, Berry EM. Diet and disease--the Israeli paradox: possible dangers of a high omega-6 polyunsaturated fatty acid diet. Isr J Med Sci. 1996 Nov;32(11):1134-43. PMID: 8960090.

22. Shapira N. Israeli 'cancer shift' over heart disease mortality may be led by greater risk in women with high intake of n-6 fatty acids. Eur J Cancer Prev. 2007 Oct;16(5):486-94. doi:

10.1097/CEJ.0b013e3280145b6d. PMID: 17923822.

23. Morton Lee Pearce et al, Incidence of cancer in men on a diet high in polyunsaturated fats, The Lancet.

24. Michel de Lorgeril, New insights into the health effects of dietary saturated and omega-6 and omega-3 polyunsaturated fatty acids, BMC Medicine201210:50, DOI: 10.1186/1741- 7015-10-50, de Lorgeril and Salen; licensee BioMed Central Ltd. 2012, Received: 17 February 2012, Accepted: 21 May 2012, Published: 21 May 2012.

25. Gago-Dominguez M, Yuan JM, Sun CL, Lee HP, Yu MC., Opposing effects of dietary n-3 and n-6 fatty acids on mammary carcinogenesis: The Singapore Chinese Health Study., Br J Cancer. 2003 Nov 3;89(9):1686-92.

26. Murff HJ, Shu XO, Li H, Yang G, Wu X, Cai H, Wen W, Gao YT, Zheng W., Dietary polyunsaturated fatty acids and breast cancer risk in Chinese women: a prospective cohort study., Int J Cancer. 2011 Mar 15;128(6):1434-41. doi: 10.1002/ijc.25703. Epub 2010 Nov 23.

27. Chajès V, Torres-Mejía G, Biessy C, Ortega-Olvera C, Angeles-Llerenas A, Ferrari P, Lazcano-Ponce E, Romieu I., ω-3 and ω-6 Polyunsaturated fatty acid intakes and the risk of breast cancer in Mexican women: impact of obesity status., Cancer Epidemiol Biomarkers Prev. 2012 Feb;21(2):319-26. doi: 10.1158/1055-9965.EPI-11-0896. Epub 2011 Dec 22.

28. Neal Simonsen , Pieter van't Veer , John J. Strain , José M. Martin-Moreno, Jussi K. Huttunen, Joaquin Femández-Crehuet Navajas, Blaise C. Martin, Michael Thamm, Alwine F. M. Kardinaal, Frans J. Kok and Lenore Kohlmeier, Adipose Tissue Omega-3 and Omega-6 Fatty Acid Content and Breast Cancer in the EURAMIC Study, Am. J. Epidemiol. (1998) 147 (4): 342-352.

29. Sonestedt E , Ericson U, Gullberg B, Skog K, Olsson H, Wirfält E., Do both heterocyclic amines and omega-6 polyunsaturated fatty acids contribute to the incidence of breast cancer in postmenopausal women of the Malmö diet and cancer cohort? , Int J Cancer. 2008 Oct 1;123(7):1637-43. doi: 10.1002/ijc.23394.

30. Petroski W, Minich DM. Is There Such a Thing as "Anti-Nutrients"? A Narrative Review of Perceived Problematic Plant Compounds. Nutrients. 2020 Sep 24;12(10):2929. doi: 10.3390/nu12102929. PMID: 32987890; PMCID: PMC7600777.

Chapter 3

1. Katarina Melzer (2011). Carbohydrate and fat utilization during rest

and physical activity. , 6(2), 0–. doi:10.1016/j.eclnm.2011.01.005

2. Boden G. Effects of free fatty acids (FFA) on glucose metabolism: significance for insulin resistance and type 2 diabetes. Exp Clin Endocrinol Diabetes. 2003 May;111(3):121-4. doi: 10.1055/s-2003-39781. PMID: 12784183.

3. DiPalma JR, Thayer WS. Use of niacin as a drug. Annu Rev Nutr. 1991;11:169-87. doi: 10.1146/annurev.nu.11.070191.001125. PMID: 1832551.

4. Lucidi P, Rossetti P, Porcellati F, Pampanelli S, Candeloro P, Andreoli AM, Perriello G, Bolli GB, Fanelli CG. Mechanisms of insulin resistance after insulin-induced hypoglycemia in humans: the role of lipolysis. Diabetes. 2010 Jun;59(6):1349-57. doi: 10.2337/db09-0745. Epub 2010 Mar 18. PMID: 20299466; PMCID: PMC2874695.

5. RANDLE PJ, GARLAND PB, HALES CN, NEWSHOLME EA. The glucose fatty-acid cycle. Its role in insulin sensitivity and the metabolic disturbances of diabetes mellitus. Lancet. 1963 Apr 13;1(7285):785-9. doi: 10.1016/s0140-6736(63)91500-9. PMID: 13990765.

6. Saponaro C, Gaggini M, Carli F, Gastaldelli A. The Subtle Balance between Lipolysis and Lipogenesis: A Critical Point in Metabolic Homeostasis. Nutrients. 2015 Nov 13;7(11):9453-74. doi: 10.3390/nu7115475. PMID: 26580649; PMCID: PMC4663603.

7. Cotter TG, Rinella M. Nonalcoholic Fatty Liver Disease 2020: The State of the Disease. Gastroenterology. 2020 May;158(7):1851-1864. doi: 10.1053/j.gastro.2020.01.052. Epub 2020 Feb 13. PMID: 32061595.

8. Lee DH, Jacobs DR Jr, Lind L, Lind PM. Lipophilic Environmental Chemical Mixtures Released During Weight-Loss: The Need to Consider Dynamics. Bioessays. 2020 Jun;42(6):e1900237. doi: 10.1002/bies.201900237. Epub 2020 May 4. PMID: 32363609.

9. Mitrakou A, Ryan C, Veneman T, Mokan M, Jenssen T, Kiss I, Durrant J, Cryer P, Gerich J. Hierarchy of glycemic thresholds for counterregulatory hormone secretion, symptoms, and cerebral dysfunction. Am J Physiol. 1991 Jan;260(1 Pt 1):E67-74. doi: 10.1152/ajpendo.1991.260.1.E67. PMID: 1987794.

10. Fowelin J, Attvall S, Von Schenck H, Smith U, Lager I. Combined effect of growth hormone and cortisol on late posthypoglycemic insulin resistance in humans. Diabetes. 1989 Nov;38(11):1357-64. doi: 10.2337/diab.38.11.1357. PMID: 2576005.

11. Vogelzangs N, Beekman AT, Milaneschi Y, Bandinelli S, Ferrucci L, Penninx BW. Urinary cortisol and six-year risk of all-cause and cardiovascular mortality. J Clin Endocrinol Metab. 2010

Nov;95(11):4959-64. doi: 10.1210/jc.2010-0192. Epub 2010 Aug 25. PMID: 20739384; PMCID: PMC2968721.

12. Reuben DB, Talvi SL, Rowe JW, Seeman TE. High urinary catecholamine excretion predicts mortality and functional decline in high-functioning, community-dwelling older persons: MacArthur Studies of Successful Aging. J Gerontol A Biol Sci Med Sci. 2000 Oct;55(10):M618-24. doi: 10.1093/gerona/55.10.m618. PMID: 11034236.

13. Covarrubias, A.J., Perrone, R., Grozio, A. et al. NAD+ metabolism and its roles in cellular processes during ageing. Nat Rev Mol Cell Biol 22, 119–141 (2021). https://doi.org/10.1038/s41580-020-00313-x

14. Xue Y, Shamp T, Nagana Gowda GA, Crabtree M, Bagchi D, Raftery D. A Combination of Nicotinamide and D-Ribose (RiaGev) Is Safe and Effective to Increase NAD+ Metabolome in Healthy Middle-Aged Adults: A Randomized, Triple-Blind, Placebo-Controlled, Cross-Over Pilot Clinical Trial. Nutrients. 2022 May 26;14(11):2219. doi: 10.3390/nu14112219. PMID: 35684021; PMCID: PMC9183138.

15. DiPalma JR, Thayer WS. Use of niacin as a drug. Annu Rev Nutr. 1991;11:169-87. doi: 10.1146/annurev.nu.11.070191.001125. PMID: 1832551.

16. Brown WV. Niacin for lipid disorders. Indications, effectiveness, and safety. Postgrad Med. 1995 Aug;98(2):185-9, 192-3. PMID: 7630846.

17. DuBroff R, de Lorgeril M. Cholesterol confusion and statin controversy. World J Cardiol. 2015 Jul 26;7(7):404-9. doi: 10.4330/wjc.v7.i7.404. PMID: 26225201; PMCID: PMC4513492.

18. Okuyama H, Langsjoen PH, Hamazaki T, Ogushi Y, Hama R, Kobayashi T, Uchino H. Statins stimulate atherosclerosis and heart failure: pharmacological mechanisms. Expert Rev Clin Pharmacol. 2015 Mar;8(2):189-99. doi: 10.1586/17512433.2015.1011125. Epub 2015 Feb 6. Erratum in: Expert Rev Clin Pharmacol. 2015;8(4):503-5. PMID: 25655639.

19. Muldoon MF, Marsland A, Flory JD, Rabin BS, Whiteside TL, Manuck SB. Immune system differences in men with hypo- or hypercholesterolemia. Clin Immunol Immunopathol. 1997 Aug;84(2):145-9. doi: 10.1006/clin.1997.4382. PMID: 9245545.

20. Muldoon MF, Kritchevsky SB, Evans RW, Kagan VE. Serum total antioxidant activity in relative hypo- and hypercholesterolemia. Free Radic Res. 1996 Sep;25(3):239-45. doi: 10.3109/10715769609149049. PMID: 8889490.

21. U. Ravnskov, K.S. McCully, P.J. Rosch, The statin-low cholesterol-

cancer conundrum, QJM: An International Journal of Medicine, Volume 105, Issue 4, April 2012, Pages 383–388, https://doi.org/10.1093/qjmed/hcr243

22. Elias PK, Elias MF, D'Agostino RB, Sullivan LM, Wolf PA. Serum cholesterol and cognitive performance in the Framingham Heart Study. Psychosom Med. 2005 Jan-Feb;67(1):24-30. doi: 10.1097/01.psy.0000151745.67285.c2. PMID: 15673620.

23. Han R. Plasma lipoproteins are important components of the immune system. Microbiol Immunol. 2010 Apr;54(4):246-53. doi: 10.1111/j.1348-0421.2010.00203.x. PMID: 20377753.

24. Weinstock C, Ullrich H, Hohe R, Berg A, Baumstark MW, Frey I, Northoff H, Flegel WA. Low density lipoproteins inhibit endotoxin activation of monocytes. Arterioscler Thromb. 1992 Mar;12(3):341-7. doi: 10.1161/01.atv.12.3.341. PMID: 1547193.

25. Flegel WA, Wölpl A, Männel DN, Northoff H. Inhibition of endotoxin-induced activation of human monocytes by human lipoproteins. Infect Immun. 1989 Jul;57(7):2237-45. doi: 10.1128/iai.57.7.2237-2245.1989. PMID: 2731990; PMCID: PMC313866.

26. Mathias Rauchhaus; Andrew JS Coats; Stefan D Anker (2000). The endotoxin-lipoprotein hypothesis., 356(9233), 0–933. doi:10.1016/s0140-6736(00)02690-8

27. Harris HW, Gosnell JE, Kumwenda ZL. The lipemia of sepsis: triglyceride-rich lipoproteins as agents of innate immunity. J Endotoxin Res. 2000;6(6):421-30. PMID: 11521066.

28. Feingold KR, Funk JL, Moser AH, Shigenaga JK, Rapp JH, Grunfeld C. Role for circulating lipoproteins in protection from endotoxin toxicity. Infect Immun. 1995 May;63(5):2041-6. doi: 10.1128/iai.63.5.2041-2046.1995. PMID: 7729918; PMCID: PMC173262.

29. Mielke MM, Zandi PP, Sjögren M, Gustafson D, Ostling S, Steen B, Skoog I. High total cholesterol levels in late life associated with a reduced risk of dementia. Neurology. 2005 May 24;64(10):1689-95. doi: 10.1212/01.WNL.0000161870.78572.A5. PMID: 15911792.

30. Weverling-Rijnsburger AW, Blauw GJ, Lagaay AM, Knook DL, Meinders AE, Westendorp RG. Total cholesterol and risk of mortality in the oldest old. Lancet. 1997 Oct 18;350(9085):1119-23. doi: 10.1016/s0140-6736(97)04430-9. Erratum in: Lancet 1998 Jan 3;351(9095):70. PMID: 9343498.

31. Petersen LK, Christensen K, Kragstrup J. Lipid-lowering treatment to the end? A review of observational studies and RCTs on cholesterol and mortality in 80+-year olds. Age Ageing. 2010 Nov;39(6):674-80. doi: 10.1093/ageing/afq129. Epub 2010 Oct 14.

PMID: 20952373; PMCID: PMC2956535.

32. Tuikkala P, Hartikainen S, Korhonen MJ, Lavikainen P, Kettunen R, Sulkava R, Enlund H. Serum total cholesterol levels and all-cause mortality in a home-dwelling elderly population: a six-year follow-up. Scand J Prim Health Care. 2010 Jun;28(2):121-7. doi: 10.3109/02813432.2010.487371. PMID: 20470020; PMCID: PMC3442317.

33. Abrams JJ, Grundy SM. Cholesterol metabolism in hypothyroidism and hyperthyroidism in man. J Lipid Res. 1981 Feb;22(2):323-38. PMID: 7240961.

34. Feld S, Dickey RA. An Association Between Varying Degrees of Hypothyroidism and Hypercholesterolemia in Women: The Thyroid-Cholesterol Connection. Prev Cardiol. 2001 Autumn;4(4):179-182. doi: 10.1111/j.1520-037x.2001.00541.x. PMID: 11832675.

35. Kong SH, Kim JH, Park YJ, Lee JH, Hong AR, Shin CS, Cho NH. Low free T3 to free T4 ratio was associated with low muscle mass and impaired physical performance in community-dwelling aged population. Osteoporos Int. 2020 Mar;31(3):525-531. doi: 10.1007/s00198-019-05137-w. Epub 2019 Nov 29. PMID: 31784788.

36. Di Iorio, A., Paganelli, R., Abate, M. et al. Thyroid hormone signaling is associated with physical performance, muscle mass, and strength in a cohort of oldest-old: results from the Mugello study. GeroScience 43, 1053–1064 (2021). https://doi.org/10.1007/s11357-020-00302-0

Chapter 4

1. Westman EC, Mavropoulos J, Yancy WS, Volek JS. A review of low-carbohydrate ketogenic diets. Curr Atheroscler Rep. 2003 Nov;5(6):476-83. doi: 10.1007/s11883-003-0038-6. PMID: 14525681.

2. Fery F, Bourdoux P, Christophe J, Balasse EO. Hormonal and metabolic changes induced by an isocaloric isoproteinic ketogenic diet in healthy subjects. Diabete Metab. 1982 Dec;8(4):299-305. PMID: 6761185.

3. Klein S, Wolfe RR. Carbohydrate restriction regulates the adaptive response to fasting. Am J Physiol. 1992 May;262(5 Pt 1):E631-6. doi: 10.1152/ajpendo.1992.262.5.E631. PMID: 1590373.

4. Kose E, Guzel O, Demir K, Arslan N. Changes of thyroid hormonal status in patients receiving ketogenic diet due to intractable epilepsy. J Pediatr Endocrinol Metab. 2017 Apr 1;30(4):411-416. doi:

10.1515/jpem-2016-0281. PMID: 28076316.

5.   Tjepkema M, Bushnik T, Bougie E. Life expectancy of First Nations, Métis and Inuit household populations in Canada. Health Rep. 2019 Dec 18;30(12):3-10. doi: 10.25318/82-003-x201901200001-eng. PMID: 31851367.

6.   Naude CE, Brand A, Schoonees A, Nguyen KA, Chaplin M, Volmink J. Low-carbohydrate versus balanced-carbohydrate diets for reducing weight and cardiovascular risk. Cochrane Database Syst Rev. 2022 Jan 28;1(1):CD013334. doi: 10.1002/14651858.CD013334.pub2. PMID: 35088407; PMCID: PMC8795871.

7.   Hall KD, Bemis T, Brychta R, Chen KY, Courville A, Crayner EJ, Goodwin S, Guo J, Howard L, Knuth ND, Miller BV 3rd, Prado CM, Siervo M, Skarulis MC, Walter M, Walter PJ, Yannai L. Calorie for Calorie, Dietary Fat Restriction Results in More Body Fat Loss than Carbohydrate Restriction in People with Obesity. Cell Metab. 2015 Sep 1;22(3):427-36. doi: 10.1016/j.cmet.2015.07.021. Epub 2015 Aug 13. PMID: 26278052; PMCID: PMC4603544.

8.   Hill, J O; Prentice, A M (1995). Sugar and body weight regulation. The American Journal of Clinical Nutrition, 62(1), 264S–273S. doi:10.1093/ajcn/62.1.264S

9.   Gheibi S, Kashfi K, Ghasemi A. A practical guide for induction of type-2 diabetes in rat: Incorporating a high-fat diet and streptozotocin. Biomed Pharmacother. 2017 Nov;95:605-613. doi: 10.1016/j.biopha.2017.08.098. Epub 2017 Sep 4. PMID: 28881291.

10. Cipryan L, Maffetone PB, Plews DJ, Laursen PB. Effects of a four-week very low-carbohydrate high-fat diet on biomarkers of inflammation: Non-randomised parallel-group study. Nutrition and Health. 2020;26(1):35-42. doi:10.1177/0260106020903206

11. Whittaker J, Harris M. Low-carbohydrate diets and men's cortisol and testosterone: Systematic review and meta-analysis. Nutr Health. 2022 Dec;28(4):543-554. doi: 10.1177/02601060221083079. Epub 2022 Mar 7. Erratum in: Nutr Health. 2022 Dec;28(4):783. PMID: 35254136; PMCID: PMC9716400.

12. Cumming DC, Quigley ME, Yen SS. Acute suppression of circulating testosterone levels by cortisol in men. J Clin Endocrinol Metab. 1983 Sep;57(3):671-3. doi: 10.1210/jcem-57-3-671. PMID: 6348068.

13. Nimgampalle, Mallikarjuna (2021). Recent Developments in Applied Microbiology and Biochemistry || Glucose metabolism in the brain: An update., (), 77–88. doi:10.1016/B978-0-12-821406-0.00008-4

14. Horton TJ, Drougas H, Brachey A, Reed GW, Peters JC, Hill JO.

185

Fat and carbohydrate overfeeding in humans: different effects on energy storage. Am J Clin Nutr. 1995 Jul;62(1):19-29. doi: 10.1093/ajcn/62.1.19. PMID: 7598063.

15. Mergenthaler P, Lindauer U, Dienel GA, Meisel A. Sugar for the brain: the role of glucose in physiological and pathological brain function. Trends Neurosci. 2013 Oct;36(10):587-97. doi: 10.1016/j.tins.2013.07.001. Epub 2013 Aug 20. PMID: 23968694; PMCID: PMC3900881.

Chapter 5

1. Noni L. Bodkin, Theresa M. Alexander, Heidi K. Ortmeyer, Elizabeth Johnson, Barbara C. Hansen, Mortality and Morbidity in Laboratory-maintained Rhesus Monkeys and Effects of Long-term Dietary Restriction, The Journals of Gerontology: Series A, Volume 58, Issue 3, March 2003, Pages B212–B219, https://doi.org/10.1093/gerona/58.3.B212

2. Soeters MR, Lammers NM, Dubbelhuis PF, Ackermans M, Jonkers-Schuitema CF, Fliers E, Sauerwein HP, Aerts JM, Serlie MJ. Intermittent fasting does not affect whole-body glucose, lipid, or protein metabolism. Am J Clin Nutr. 2009 Nov;90(5):1244-51. doi: 10.3945/ajcn.2008.27327. Epub 2009 Sep 23. PMID: 19776143.

3. Lowe DA, Wu N, Rohdin-Bibby L, et al. Effects of Time-Restricted Eating on Weight Loss and Other Metabolic Parameters in Women and Men With Overweight and Obesity: The TREAT Randomized Clinical Trial. JAMA Intern Med. 2020;180(11):1491–1499. doi:10.1001/jamainternmed.2020.4153

4. https://www.cnbc.com/2020/09/28/intermittent-fasting-doesnt-help-weight-loss-ucsf-study.html; Retrieved 20th November 2023.

5. Cienfuegos S, Corapi S, Gabel K, Ezpeleta M, Kalam F, Lin S, Pavlou V, Varady KA. Effect of Intermittent Fasting on Reproductive Hormone Levels in Females and Males: A Review of Human Trials. Nutrients. 2022 Jun 3;14(11):2343. doi: 10.3390/nu14112343.

6. Moro T, Tinsley G, Pacelli FQ, Marcolin G, Bianco A, Paoli A. Twelve Months of Time-restricted Eating and Resistance Training Improves Inflammatory Markers and Cardiometabolic Risk Factors. Med Sci Sports Exerc. 2021 Dec 1;53(12):2577-2585. doi: 10.1249/MSS.0000000000002738. PMID: 34649266; PMCID: PMC10115489.

7. Moro T, Tinsley G, Bianco A, Marcolin G, Pacelli QF, Battaglia G, Palma A, Gentil P, Neri M, Paoli A. Effects of eight weeks of time-

186

restricted feeding (16/8) on basal metabolism, maximal strength, body composition, inflammation, and cardiovascular risk factors in resistance-trained males. J Transl Med. 2016 Oct 13;14(1):290. doi: 10.1186/s12967-016-1044-0. PMID: 27737674; PMCID: PMC5064803.

8. Michalsen, A. Prolonged Fasting as a Method of Mood Enhancement in Chronic Pain Syndromes: A Review of Clinical Evidence and Mechanisms. Curr Pain Headache Rep 14, 80–87 (2010). https://doi.org/10.1007/s11916-010-0104-z

9. Bergendahl M, Vance ML, Iranmanesh A, Thorner MO, Veldhuis JD. Fasting as a metabolic stress paradigm selectively amplifies cortisol secretory burst mass and delays the time of maximal nyctohemeral cortisol concentrations in healthy men. J Clin Endocrinol Metab. 1996 Feb;81(2):692-9. doi: 10.1210/jcem.81.2.8636290. PMID: 8636290.

10. Boelen A, Wiersinga WM, Fliers E. Fasting-induced changes in the hypothalamus-pituitary-thyroid axis. Thyroid. 2008 Feb;18(2):123-9. doi: 10.1089/thy.2007.0253. PMID: 18225975.

11. Laurens C, Grundler F, Damiot A, Chery I, Le Maho AL, Zahariev A, Le Maho Y, Bergouignan A, Gauquelin-Koch G, Simon C, Blanc S, Wilhelmi de Toledo F. Is muscle and protein loss relevant in long-term fasting in healthy men? A prospective trial on physiological adaptations. J Cachexia Sarcopenia Muscle. 2021 Dec;12(6):1690-1703. doi: 10.1002/jcsm.12766. Epub 2021 Oct 20. PMID: 34668663; PMCID: PMC8718030.

12. Letkiewicz S, Pilis K, Ślęzak A, Pilis A, Pilis W, Żychowska M, Langfort J. Eight Days of Water-Only Fasting Promotes Favorable Changes in the Functioning of the Urogenital System of Middle-Aged Healthy Men. Nutrients. 2020 Dec 30;13(1):113. doi: 10.3390/nu13010113. PMID: 33396948; PMCID: PMC7824351.

13. Egas Moniz – Facts. NobelPrize.org. Nobel Prize Outreach AB 2023. Sat. 9 Dec 2023. https://www.nobelprize.org/prizes/medicine/1949/moniz/facts

14. Gump JM, Thorburn A. Autophagy and apoptosis: what is the connection? Trends Cell Biol. 2011 Jul;21(7):387-92. doi: 10.1016/j.tcb.2011.03.007. Epub 2011 May 10. PMID: 21561772; PMCID: PMC3539742.

15. Vargas, J.N.S., Hamasaki, M., Kawabata, T. et al. The mechanisms and roles of selective autophagy in mammals. Nat Rev Mol Cell Biol 24, 167–185 (2023). https://doi.org/10.1038/s41580-022-00542-2

16. He C, Bassik MC, Moresi V, Sun K, Wei Y, Zou Z, An Z, Loh J, Fisher J, Sun Q, Korsmeyer S, Packer M, May HI, Hill JA, Virgin

HW, Gilpin C, Xiao G, Bassel-Duby R, Scherer PE, Levine B. Exercise-induced BCL2-regulated autophagy is required for muscle glucose homeostasis. Nature. 2012 Jan 18;481(7382):511-5. doi: 10.1038/nature10758. Erratum in: Nature. 2013 Nov 7:503(7474):146. PMID: 22258505; PMCID: PMC3518436.

17. Speakman JR, Hambly C. Starving for life: what animal studies can and cannot tell us about the use of caloric restriction to prolong human lifespan. J Nutr. 2007 Apr;137(4):1078-86. doi: 10.1093/jn/137.4.1078. PMID: 17374682.

18. López-Domínguez JA, Ramsey JJ, Tran D, Imai DM, Koehne A, Laing ST, Griffey SM, Kim K, Taylor SL, Hagopian K, Villalba JM, López-Lluch G, Navas P, McDonald RB. The Influence of Dietary Fat Source on Life Span in Calorie Restricted Mice. J Gerontol A Biol Sci Med Sci. 2015 Oct;70(10):1181-8. doi: 10.1093/gerona/glu177. Epub 2014 Oct 13. PMID: 25313149; PMCID: PMC4612357.

19. Villareal DT, Fontana L, Das SK, Redman L, Smith SR, Saltzman E, Bales C, Rochon J, Pieper C, Huang M, Lewis M, Schwartz AV; CALERIE Study Group. Effect of Two-Year Caloric Restriction on Bone Metabolism and Bone Mineral Density in Non-Obese Younger Adults: A Randomized Clinical Trial. J Bone Miner Res. 2016 Jan;31(1):40-51. doi: 10.1002/jbmr.2701. Epub 2015 Sep 24. PMID: 26332798; PMCID: PMC4834845.

20. Alharbi TA, Paudel S, Gasevic D, Ryan J, Freak-Poli R, Owen AJ. The association of weight change and all-cause mortality in older adults: a systematic review and meta-analysis. Age Ageing. 2021 May 5;50(3):697-704. doi: 10.1093/ageing/afaa231. PMID: 33161429.

21. Cheng FW, Gao X, Jensen GL. Weight Change and All-Cause Mortality in Older Adults: A Meta-Analysis. J Nutr Gerontol Geriatr. 2015;34(4):343-68. doi: 10.1080/21551197.2015.1090362. PMID: 26571354.

22. Chen C, Ye Y, Zhang Y, Pan XF, Pan A. Weight change across adulthood in relation to all cause and cause specific mortality: prospective cohort study. BMJ. 2019 Oct 16;367:l5584. doi: 10.1136/bmj.l5584. PMID: 31619383; PMCID: PMC6812615.

23. Alharbi T, Ryan J, Freak-Poli R, Gasevic D, Scali J, Ritchie K, Ancelin ML, Owen AJ. Objectively Assessed Weight Change and All-Cause Mortality among Community-Dwelling Older People. Nutrients. 2022 Jul 21;14(14):2983. doi: 10.3390/nu14142983. PMID: 35889940; PMCID: PMC9320907.

24. Hussain SM, Newman AB, Beilin LJ, Tonkin AM, Woods RL, Neumann JT, Nelson M, Carr PR, Reid CM, Owen A, Ball J, Cicut-

tini FM, Tran C, Wang Y, Ernst ME, McNeil JJ. Associations of Change in Body Size With All-Cause and Cause-Specific Mortality Among Healthy Older Adults. JAMA Netw Open. 2023 Apr 3;6(4):e237482. doi: 10.1001/jamanetworkopen.2023.7482. PMID: 37036703; PMCID: PMC10087052.

25. Andres R, Muller DC, Sorkin JD. Long-term effects of change in body weight on all-cause mortality. A review. Ann Intern Med. 1993 Oct 1;119(7 Pt 2):737-43. doi: 10.7326/0003-4819-119-7_part_2-199310011-00022. PMID: 8363208.

26. Lee DH, Jacobs DR Jr, Lind L, Lind PM. Lipophilic Environmental Chemical Mixtures Released During Weight-Loss: The Need to Consider Dynamics. Bioessays. 2020 Jun;42(6):e1900237. doi: 10.1002/bies.201900237. Epub 2020 May 4. PMID: 32363609.

27. Yancy WS Jr, Olsen MK, Guyton JR, Bakst RP, Westman EC. A low-carbohydrate, ketogenic diet versus a low-fat diet to treat obesity and hyperlipidemia: a randomized, controlled trial. Ann Intern Med. 2004 May 18;140(10):769-77. doi: 10.7326/0003-4819-140-10-200405180-00006. PMID: 15148063.

28. Flegal KM, Kit BK, Orpana H, Graubard BI. Association of all-cause mortality with overweight and obesity using standard body mass index categories: a systematic review and meta-analysis. JAMA. 2013 Jan 2;309(1):71-82. doi: 10.1001/jama.2012.113905. PMID: 23280227; PMCID: PMC4855514.

29. Lennon H, Sperrin M, Badrick E, Renehan AG. The Obesity Paradox in Cancer: a Review. Curr Oncol Rep. 2016 Sep;18(9):56. doi: 10.1007/s11912-016-0539-4. PMID: 27475805; PMCID: PMC4967417.

30. Carnethon MR, De Chavez PJ, Biggs ML, Lewis CE, Pankow JS, Bertoni AG, Golden SH, Liu K, Mukamal KJ, Campbell-Jenkins B, Dyer AR. Association of weight status with mortality in adults with incident diabetes. JAMA. 2012 Aug 8;308(6):581-90. doi: 10.1001/jama.2012.9282. Erratum in: JAMA. 2012 Nov 28;308(20):2085. PMID: 22871870; PMCID: PMC3467944.

Chapter 6

1. Morgan CA 3rd, Hazlett G, Southwick S, Rasmusson A, Lieberman HR. Effect of carbohydrate administration on recovery from stress-induced deficits in cognitive function: a double-blind, placebo-controlled study of soldiers exposed to survival school stress. Mil Med. 2009 Feb;174(2):132-8. doi: 10.7205/milmed-d-58-7808. PMID: 19317193.

2.   Bruni O, Ferini-Strambi L, Giacomoni E, Pellegrino P. Herbal Remedies and Their Possible Effect on the GABAergic System and Sleep. Nutrients. 2021 Feb 6;13(2):530. doi: 10.3390/nu13020530. PMID: 33561990; PMCID: PMC7914492.

3.   Byun JI, Shin YY, Chung SE, Shin WC. Safety and Efficacy of Gamma-Aminobutyric Acid from Fermented Rice Germ in Patients with Insomnia Symptoms: A Randomized, Double-Blind Trial.   J   Clin   Neurol.   2018   Jul;14(3):291-295.   doi: 10.3988/jcn.2018.14.3.291. Epub 2018 Apr 27. PMID: 29856155; PMCID: PMC6031986.

4.   Chen S, Kang J, Zhu H, Wang K, Han Z, Wang L, Liu J, Wu Y, He P, Tu Y, Li B. L-Theanine and Immunity: A Review. Molecules. 2023 May 1;28(9):3846. doi: 10.3390/molecules28093846. PMID: 37175254; PMCID: PMC10179891.

5.   Williams JL, Everett JM, D'Cunha NM, Sergi D, Georgousopoulou EN, Keegan RJ, McKune AJ, Mellor DD, Anstice N, Naumovski N. The Effects of Green Tea Amino Acid L-Theanine Consumption on the Ability to Manage Stress and Anxiety Levels: a Systematic Review. Plant Foods Hum Nutr. 2020 Mar;75(1):12-23. doi: 10.1007/s11130-019-00771-5. PMID: 31758301.

6.   Lopes Sakamoto F, Metzker Pereira Ribeiro R, Amador Bueno A, Oliveira Santos H. Psychotropic effects of L-theanine and its clinical properties: From the management of anxiety and stress to a potential use in schizophrenia. Pharmacol Res. 2019 Sep;147:104395. doi: 10.1016/j.phrs.2019.104395. Epub 2019 Aug 11. PMID: 31412272.

7.   Powell JG, Garland S, Preston K, Piszczatoski C. Brexanolone (Zulresso): Finally, an FDA-Approved Treatment for Postpartum Depression. Ann Pharmacother. 2020 Feb;54(2):157-163. doi: 10.1177/1060028019873320. Epub 2019 Sep 3. PMID: 31476884.

8.   https://www.psycom.net/mental-health-medications/brexanalone; Retrieved 20th nov 2023

9.   Boero G, Porcu P, Morrow AL. Pleiotropic actions of allopregnanolone underlie therapeutic benefits in stress-related disease. Neurobiol   Stress.   2019   Nov   27;12:100203.   doi: 10.1016/j.ynstr.2019.100203.   PMID: 31879693;   PMCID: PMC6920111.

10.   Milivojevic V, Sullivan L, Tiber J, Fogelman N, Simpson C, Hermes G, Sinha R. Pregnenolone effects on provoked alcohol craving, anxiety, HPA axis, and autonomic arousal in individuals with alcohol use disorder. Psychopharmacology (Berl). 2023 Jan;240(1):101-114. doi: 10.1007/s00213-022-06278-3. Epub 2022 Nov 29. PMID: 36445398; PMCID: PMC10630889.

11. Milivojevic V, Charron L, Fogelman N, Hermes G, Sinha R. Pregnenolone Reduces Stress-Induced Craving, Anxiety, and Autonomic Arousal in Individuals with Cocaine Use Disorder. Biomolecules. 2022 Oct 29;12(11):1593. doi: 10.3390/biom12111593. PMID: 36358943; PMCID: PMC9687893.

12. Milivojevic V, Fox HC, Sofuoglu M, Covault J, Sinha R. Effects of progesterone stimulated allopregnanolone on craving and stress response in cocaine dependent men and women. Psychoneuroendocrinology. 2016 Mar;65:44-53. doi: 10.1016/j.psyneuen.2015.12.008. Epub 2015 Dec 14. PMID: 26716877; PMCID: PMC4752896.

Chapter 7

1. Brown GC. The endotoxin hypothesis of neurodegeneration. J Neuroinflammation. 2019 Sep 13;16(1):180. doi: 10.1186/s12974-019-1564-7. PMID: 31519175; PMCID: PMC6744684.

2. Mehta NN, McGillicuddy FC, Anderson PD, Hinkle CC, Shah R, Pruscino L, Tabita-Martinez J, Sellers KF, Rickels MR, Reilly MP. Experimental endotoxemia induces adipose inflammation and insulin resistance in humans. Diabetes. 2010 Jan;59(1):172-81. doi: 10.2337/db09-0367. Epub 2009 Sep 30. PMID: 19794059; PMCID: PMC2797919.

3. Lassenius, M. I. et al. Bacterial endotoxin activity in human serum is associated with dyslipidemia, insulin resistance, obesity, and chronic inflammation. Diabetes Care 34, 1809–15 (2011).

4. Carnevale, R., Nocella, C., Petrozza, V. et al. Localization of lipopolysaccharide from Escherichia Coli into human atherosclerotic plaque. Sci Rep 8, 3598 (2018). https://doi.org/10.1038/s41598-018-22076-4

5. Wong VW, Wong GL, Chan HY, Yeung DK, Chan RS, Chim AM, Chan CK, Tse YK, Woo J, Chu WC, Chan HL. Bacterial endotoxin and non-alcoholic fatty liver disease in the general population: a prospective cohort study. Aliment Pharmacol Ther. 2015 Sep;42(6):731-40. doi: 10.1111/apt.13327. Epub 2015 Jul 23. PMID: 26202818.

6. Harte AL, da Silva NF, Creely SJ, McGee KC, Billyard T, Youssef-Elabd EM, Tripathi G, Ashour E, Abdalla MS, Sharada HM, Amin AI, Burt AD, Kumar S, Day CP, McTernan PG. Elevated endotoxin levels in non-alcoholic fatty liver disease. J Inflamm (Lond). 2010 Mar 30;7:15. doi: 10.1186/1476-9255-7-15. PMID: 20353583; PMCID: PMC2873499.

7. Gomes JMG, Costa JA, Alfenas RCG. Metabolic endotoxemia and

diabetes mellitus: A systematic review. Metabolism. 2017 Mar;68:133-144. doi: 10.1016/j.metabol.2016.12.009. Epub 2016 Dec 18. PMID: 28183445.

8. Stehle JR Jr, Leng X, Kitzman DW, Nicklas BJ, Kritchevsky SB, High KP. Lipopolysaccharide-binding protein, a surrogate marker of microbial translocation, is associated with physical function in healthy older adults. J Gerontol A Biol Sci Med Sci. 2012 Nov;67(11):1212-8. doi: 10.1093/gerona/gls178. Epub 2012 Sep 7. PMID: 22960476; PMCID: PMC3636679.

9. O'Dwyer ST, Michie HR, Ziegler TR, Revhaug A, Smith RJ, Wilmore DW. A Single Dose of Endotoxin Increases Intestinal Permeability in Healthy Humans. Arch Surg. 1988;123(12):1459–1464. doi:10.1001/archsurg.1988.01400360029003

10. Guo S, Al-Sadi R, Said HM, Ma TY. Lipopolysaccharide causes an increase in intestinal tight junction permeability in vitro and in vivo by inducing enterocyte membrane expression and localization of TLR-4 and CD14. Am J Pathol. 2013 Feb;182(2):375-87. doi: 10.1016/j.ajpath.2012.10.014. Epub 2012 Nov 29. PMID: 23201091; PMCID: PMC3562736.

11. Ho, Kok-Sun (2012). Stopping or reducing dietary fiber intake reduces constipation and its associated symptoms. World Journal of Gastroenterology, 18(33), 4593–. doi:10.3748/wjg.v18.i33.4593

12. Balan I, Patterson R, Boero G, Krohn H, O'Buckley TK, Meltzer-Brody S, Morrow AL. Brexanolone therapeutics in post-partum depression involves inhibition of systemic inflammatory pathways. EBioMedicine. 2023 Mar;89:104473. doi: 10.1016/j.ebiom.2023.104473. Epub 2023 Feb 16. PMID: 36801618; PMCID: PMC9984433.

13. Boero G, Porcu P, Morrow AL. Pleiotropic actions of allopregnanolone underlie therapeutic benefits in stress-related disease. Neurobiol Stress. 2019 Nov 27;12:100203. doi: 10.1016/j.ynstr.2019.100203. PMID: 31879693; PMCID: PMC6920111.

14. Metabolic Effects of Intermittent Fasting Ruth E. Patterson and Dorothy D. Sears Annual Review of Nutrition 2017 37:1, 371-393

Made in the USA
Columbia, SC
27 February 2025